ENERGETIC DIAGNOSIS

How to evaluate patients' PERSONAL ENERGIES using INTUITION and NEW MEDICAL DEVICES to improve our ability to diagnose and treat COMPLEX MEDICAL ILLNESSES

Neil Nathan, MD

VICTORY BELT PUBLISHING
LAS VEGAS

TABLE OF CONTENTS

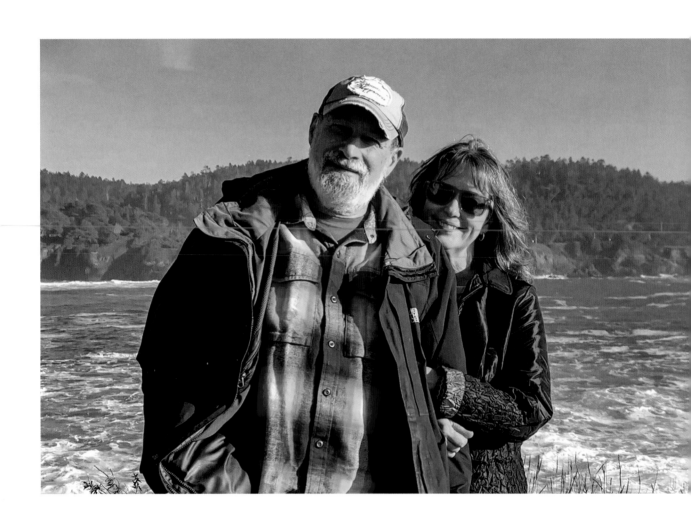

DEDICATION

GREET, PRAY, LOVE: Our Recipe for Nurturing and Sustaining Love

I said after the last book that I wouldn't dedicate my next book to my magical Cheryl, but how could I not?

The most sacred, special, enchanted moment of my day is when I hold my beloved Cheryl. We have created a kind of ritual around this holding. I get up a bit earlier than she does, and, after kissing her shoulder or back upon arising, I go into the kitchen and make coffee (after feeding the cat, turning up the heat in the house, and letting our dogs, Joey and Sasha, out). I bring her a cup of coffee, which she sips slowly as she wakes up, and then she comes into the kitchen for our embrace. I sit on a barstool and she nestles up to me. This creates a connection in which I can feel every part of her body snuggle into mine; we fit perfectly. As I savor this perfect moment, I am transported into a deeply appreciative, blissful state. I feel so nourished, so cherished, and so lucky that we can enjoy this embrace, which lasts anywhere from a few seconds to a minute or two. Although this is only a moment in time, I know, somewhere in the essence of my being, that this is the true experience of love.

Taking the time to do this every single day, as a ritual, reinforces our commitment to each other and to the importance of how we connect on every level. Words need not be spoken. As we are both strongly kinesthetic, it is our touch that binds us, again, to enjoy yet another day that we have to spend together. No matter what happens later, we have this moment; this unspoken sharing that sets the tone for a new day of perfect connection, which we endeavor to re-create as often as possible as the day evolves.

A Return to Our Birthright

MEDICAL CARE
IS NOT WHAT IT USED TO BE.

When I was growing up, a general practitioner took care of our whole family. He knew all of us and was almost always available to attend to our medical needs. For most of us today, we may or may not know the person we see for our medical care. That person is likely to keep their back turned to us for the duration of our seven-minute appointment while they type information into a digital record. And if you call the office with a medical question, the staff may not get back to you for several weeks. Yes, there are wonderful exceptions, but for the most part, this is what modern medicine has evolved into. How did this come to pass?

In the late 1940s, with the arrival of antibiotics and vaccines, we were promised that the end of infectious disease was just around the corner. We were promised that the latest technologies combined with medical science were going to make illness a thing of the past.

Alas, we were misled. The microbes were far more intelligent and communicative than we realized and developed resistance to those antibiotics faster than we could develop new drugs. Our vaccines do not live up to their promises (with a few exceptions), yet they are promoted as critical to our health. For example, the flu vaccine is prepared in the spring, before the arrival in the fall of the next wave of a mutated virus that will create our next epidemic. There are approximately 3,000 strains of flu virus, and the vaccine is made against just four of those strains; these are the ones that the Centers for Disease Control (CDC), World Health Organization (WHO), and other collaborating medical facilities think will infect the most people in the coming season. A rough calculation shows us that there is a 1 in 1,000 chance that the CDC will guess correctly.

With the exception of H1N1, for which there was eighteen months of lead time, they have not made the correct predictions yet.

One of the most common causes of death in Americans is side effects from medications, and another is health complications during hospital stays.

Please don't get me wrong: I would not be alive today but for my five-day stay in a wonderful hospital with intravenous antibiotics and the intervention of a superb colorectal surgeon. For that I will be forever grateful. But somewhere along the line, we have lost our way. The physicians of the past and the native healers, without these technologies, were able to successfully treat many of the ailments that they attended to. In our current arrogance, we dismiss this as primitive.

Those healers took the time to get to know the folks who came to them for assistance and had learned, over many years of apprenticeship and study, to read the energies of those folks and help them. They did not have access to the wonderful technologies we do now. MRI scans, CAT scans, and PET scans can show us, with a fair amount of precision, what is going on inside the body. In our not-so-distant past, without those tools, native healers, shamans, medicine men, and physicians used their perceptual gifts, refined over many years of study and training, to relieve the pain and suffering of those who came to them for help. While many may view these administrations as primitive, they must have been somewhat successful, for we, as their descendants, are here to continue their lineage.

Given our love for new technologies and our increasingly limited time spent with patients, many physicians rely so completely on scans and tests that it is rare for a specialist (for example, an orthopedist or neurosurgeon) who is evaluating a patient with pain to examine that patient in anything beyond a cursory manner. Having been a pain specialist myself for thirty-plus years, most of the patients referred to me said that I was the first physician to physically examine them. Our reliance on technology has, in many ways, distanced us from the beings who come to us for healing. We are placing less and less value on the abilities to listen to and touch our patients and, accordingly, are overlooking a wealth of important information that we need to diagnose what is wrong with them.

Those who preceded us in the distant past were able to take in a great deal of information by spending time with their patients. Let's use the simple example of "taking the pulse"—an apt term. Most physicians, who will be making the diagnosis, no longer take their patients' pulses. Nurses handle this task and simply chart the number of beats per minute. It's a simple thing, but of course there is more. Is the pulse strong, steady, or weak (thready)? Does it speak of vitality or weakness? A moment of touching the wrist to feel the pulse can tell us a lot about a person, if we do it. (Later, in the chapter on acupuncture, I will talk a great deal more about that.)

In this way, we begin to get in touch with the energy system of our patient. In medicine today, we do not talk much about energy. And yet we are energetic beings: we constantly radiate the energies of our many biological systems out into the world, which can be appreciated by those who make the effort to perceive those energies. Think about it: The heart has an electrical system that coordinates the beating of the different chambers so that blood flows smoothly to all parts of the body that need it. We measure that electrical activity with an electrocardiogram (EKG), which is a basic tool of medicine. Likewise, the brain radiates brain waves constantly, and we measure those waves with an electroencephalogram (EEG).

These are the most obvious examples of the parts of our bodies that generate electromagnetic fields. So why would it take a leap of faith to understand that just as the ears are capable of taking in sound waves and sending electrical signals to our brains so we can interpret those signals as music or noise or language, so, too, can we pick up other energetic signals coming in to us that we can use to appreciate other information? Our eyes take in light waves and do the same thing. Our fingers convert perceptions of touch into electrical signals that our brains interpret as painful or comfortable. Our taste buds convert biochemical signals into electrical ones that we interpret as taste. The olfactory lobes of the brain convert the scents of our environment into electrical signals that we perceive as pleasant or unpleasant.

All of our senses reflect our abilities to take in various types of stimuli and make sense of them through electrical signaling. Basically, this is energetic perception. And it is my thesis that we need to reacquire our innate gifts (not spurn them by relying solely on technology) and own and refine them in order to not only improve our ability to both diagnose and treat disease but also maximize our personal growth and our ability to interact with other beings and our environment.

This is our birthright. We are an integral part of the natural world, and we were born to live in it, take part in it, and connect to it and to those who come to us for help. That cannot be done in a seven-minute visit with your back turned to the patient, typing data into a computer. It cannot be done when your day is measured in "productivity" (translation: seeing as many patients as you can) for which you are rewarded. There is a growing recognition of an epidemic of burnout among physicians who are subjected to this kind of abuse, who are unable to help the people who come to them in need and feel overwhelmed by it all.

I would like to suggest an alternative to my colleagues and my patients. Let us own our birthright: our ability to perceive energies not yet visible to the eye or to the technologies currently in vogue. Let us in the medical field use those perceptions in the service of diagnosis and healing. That is what this book is about. It is my fervent hope that it will lead both physicians and patients back to a practice of medicine that is effective, rewarding, and most of all human.

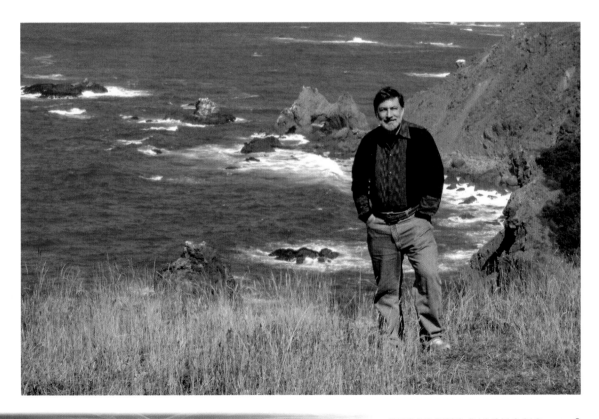

Introduction

Let me begin by explaining why I felt the need to write this book.

I have been a physician for almost fifty years. (Actually, by the time this book is in print, it will be a little over forty-nine years, but who's counting?) I began my career as a family physician who did the full gamut of medical practice: I delivered babies, did a little surgery, worked in the emergency room, admitted my patients to the hospital and followed them there, and took care of extended family systems.

What makes me a bit unusual is that I have always been especially interested in the patients I was unable to help using the tools and information I had learned in medical school. While delighted with my successes, I was drawn to study those individuals who were not improving. The foremost questions in mind were always these: What else could I learn? What new skills could I acquire that could help this patient get better? My goal, unrealistic as it might seem, has been to spend time with and help every single patient who sits down in my office.

Alas, I cannot say that I have achieved that goal, but what matters to me still, after almost five decades of trying, is that burning desire to be of service to as many patients as possible. To that end, I have tried to learn everything I can in the service of learning how to be a healer (not just a medical doctor), first by embracing conventional medical education and then adding to that base of knowledge by delving into every form of healing that seemed to have potential value.

I started this journey in medical school with a study of hypnosis, taught by one of my professors. Then, early in my medical practice when I worked in the Indian Health Service (1972), I was exposed to Native American medicine men. Going into private practice in 1974, I joined a group of interested practitioners to create a medical center that would incorporate as many types of healing as possible to be helpful to our patients. The word *holistic* had not yet come into vogue.

Over many years, I studied or incorporated into my "toolbox" a wide array of healing modalities: Reichian therapy, osteopathic manipulation (especially cranial work), therapeutic touch, acupuncture, homeopathy, Trager massage, Feldenkrais Method, and more. As overwhelming as this might seem, it progressed slowly, organically, and I learned step-by-step as I went. With each healing modality that I picked up, I was able to help more and more patients.

Later, I returned to a deeper study of biochemistry in what is now called "functional medicine," which gave me a whole set of new tools and information to help patients get better.

I have detailed this journey in two of my earlier books, *On Hope and Healing* and *Healing Is Possible,* but what I am trying to convey here is that I was passionately seeking knowledge and tools to help patients who had not received help from the conventional healthcare system. Over time, more and more colleagues began to refer their more challenging cases to me, and I slowly gained the ability to help an increasing percentage of those patients.

This leads us to where I am today. My medical practice now consists almost exclusively of patients who have been referred to me by other physicians. These patients are experiencing symptoms that they cannot explain, or are, inexplicably, unresponsive to treatments that work for other patients with the same diagnoses or symptoms. Simply put, I work with individuals who are unusually sensitive or reactive to their treatments or their environment. I welcome this challenge. It pushes me to learn more, dig deeper, and try harder to understand core questions, like "Why could I help this patient, but not that one with a seemingly identical presentation?"

At this point in my medical practice, I have helped thousands of patients with conditions that most of my colleagues do not even realize can be diagnosed and successfully treated. A few examples of these are chronic fatigue syndrome, fibromyalgia, autism, mold toxicity, Lyme disease, Alzheimer's, and autoimmune diseases.

So, after years of study, I realized that I had integrated into my practice a component of diagnosis and treatment that my colleagues were reluctant to talk about: intuition.

I pondered what had allowed me to be so successful in working with these complicated patients. I was by now recognized as a teacher, an international lecturer, and an excellent diagnostician, and I was wrestling with how to teach other healthcare providers to do what I did. Was intuition a teachable skill? Eager to answer this question, I have endeavored over the past ten years to do just that: to find out to what extent I could impart what I had learned to other physicians.

This book is a natural outgrowth of those efforts. I have come to rely on more than just my knowledge of anatomy, physiology, and biochemistry. I have learned to recognize patterns of symptoms.

When patients describe their illnesses, I listen to them with an ear to their speech, nuances, pauses, and hesitations. I try to see them with eyes that are taking in deeper layers of their presentation, such as how they are dressed and how they move, cross their legs or arms, and fidget in their chairs.

Not by intricately dissecting all of these disparate pieces of information but by sitting back and taking in the gestalt of the person sitting before me as a whole, with as much compassion and empathy as I can bring to bear, is how I have learned to do what I do. I realized that the totality of what I perceive gives me the clues I need to make a clear diagnosis of their condition, and later to help guide us to the correct treatment that will allow them to heal.

I use the word *intuition* to describe this process. But, while this word does convey an idea of what we are doing, it is more complicated than that. It is my hope that this book will provide a window for both practitioners and patients to explore, with me, the full meaning of this process. This is not, however, a how-to book. The intent is to introduce these concepts and discuss them in a personal and meaningful way. I hope it will stimulate some of my readers to acknowledge their own gifts and give them permission to explore and enhance them. If a single person is helped in this way, then this book will have been successful. (Actually, you will discover that one of my guest authors, having been given an advance copy of some of these chapters, has already had that experience.)

Over the years, it has become clear to me that a part of what we call intuition involves not only pattern recognition, which can be learned and taught, but also the perception of the energies that radiate from every human being and can be perceived by those who make the effort to cultivate the gifts we all have.

It is my belief that we are all born with innate ability to perceive these energies, but culturally most of us are taught at any early age to shun these perceptions as "unacceptable" or "weird," and we quickly suppress (but do not lose) them. It is my theory that these perceptual gifts, our birthright, need to be owned and reclaimed so that we can optimize our ability to function in this world. Given the increasing barrage of stimuli to which we are all exposed, we need these gifts to cut through this complexity and clarify our perceptions so we can operate more comfortably in our environments.

It is also my concern that now more than ever, this needs to be a priority in our personal development, because our immersion in technology is increasingly separating us from the world we live in— the natural world.

The most obvious example of this is our acceptance of virtual reality as an enjoyable substitute for the real world. As the natural world screams at us for how we are ignoring our responsibilities of taking care of this planet—by contributing to global warming, clear-cutting our forests, placing tens of thousands of new and untested chemicals into our environment, placing massive amounts of non-physiological electromagnetic fields onto planet Earth—all of the other living species on this planet are working feverishly to try to adjust. It is difficult for all of us to adjust our biochemistries quickly enough to meet these challenges, and we humans will be one of the slower species to make that change.

This is why I wrote this book: to help us understand how to honor our perceptions and bring them back into our lives in the service of healing both our individual lives and the planet that we inhabit. I called this concept *energetic diagnosis,* which can be briefly defined as the ability to recognize unique signs of illness or disease by utilizing our innate perceptual abilities.

Energetic intuition is the ability to utilize pattern recognition by trusting our conscious and subconscious perceptions to point to or provide answers to sort out seemingly complex information.

ENERGETIC INFORMATION

In-Formation: How Geese Fly and Other Forms of Alignment

Information is out there. Lots of it. Everywhere. Our eyes pick up visual information. Our ears take in auditory information. Our noses detect all sorts of smells, and our taste buds add to those perceptions when we eat. Our sense of touch is how we first connect to the universe as infants and continues to provide a constant stream of sensory input throughout our lives. Even in the womb, we begin to take in sensations and process them. Following birth, the major activities of growth and development center around refining these perceptions.

As humans evolved, we utilized the refined perception of energies to help us adjust to weather fluctuations, find food and medicinal plants, and cope with change.

Mystics of every tradition have taught us for centuries that unseen information was accessible, although only a few were able to join them perceptually. But it wasn't until the mid-1890s, when Italian inventor Guglielmo Marconi discovered how to use radio waves to conduct information over huge distances, that we embraced the reality of accessible information. Later, we learned how to transmit even more information through black-and-white images, then color television, and eventually across vast spaces so that the world could watch astronauts plant flags on the moon.

Today, even a five-year-old child knows that information can be stored, accessed, and shared through a "cloud."

So yes, it is increasingly clear that there is indeed a lot of information "out there." With a few keystrokes, I can find the name of Napoleon's brother-in-law twice removed for the crossword puzzle I am working on. I can order a cashmere sweater from a clothing store or download a book or movie in seconds.

But, as a physician and would-be healer, the information I want most is about *you*. I want to help you answer your most pressing questions, like "Why am I sick?" and "How do I get well?"

What I am getting at is that despite this vast storehouse of information located in cyberspace, often individuals do not know how to ask the right questions or where to find the right answers. The obvious source for answers to questions about your health would be you, of course. It is not likely that cyberspace has an answer that pertains to you. Yes, you can go online and peruse a list of symptoms and hope that what you are reading is going to give you answers, but in my experience, those lists are just that: lists. They cannot embrace the totality of your experiences and will most likely be incomplete.

Of course, you might get lucky. Maybe you have something simple, like a stomach virus or a thyroid hormone deficiency. However, the longer I practice medicine, the clearer it becomes that everything is connected to everything else. A long string of biochemical dominoes can come into play before you realize that you are still not feeling well. It becomes clear that a medical diagnosis isn't always accurate.

For example, let's say that your thyroid isn't working properly to produce adequate thyroid hormones. The medical paradigm is straightforward: take thyroid hormone replacement and you will be well. This kind of reliance on old information impacts the traditional medical diagnosis. While that treatment might work for some patients, the latest research shows that the inability of the thyroid to make thyroid hormones does not occur in a vacuum. What happened to set that off? (This question is rarely asked.) Did you have an autoimmune problem (the most common cause of low thyroid, or hypothyroidism), or did you experience unusual levels of stress in the form of childbirth, surgery, infection, or emotional upheaval? Were you exposed to mold or other environmental toxins, like pesticides? Was the thyroid problem triggered by other hormonal imbalances, such as adrenal stress, sex hormone deficiencies, or insulin issues, and how are all of these factors related?

The longer I practice medicine, the more I learn (and relearn) how little I know about how complicated the human body is. There are no simple questions or answers. In fact, the more we realize how little is known about the body despite hundreds of thousands of published research papers, the clearer it is that the science behind medical testing and treatment is not adequate to even begin to meet our needs. At times, even knowing where to start becomes overwhelming.

That is where intuition comes in. I have come to believe that intuition is so important, and we owe it to ourselves to recognize the power it has in our lives and learn to use it effectively.

COMING TO OUR SENSES

We are born with good sense(s). We come into this world prepared to experience this glorious universe by taking it in with all of the sensory apparatuses we bring to the table. That's how we grow, learn, and take part in this grand adventure.

We watch how an infant interacts with the world: one day, they manage to grab hold of one of those things that dangle in front of them sometimes (their foot, perhaps) and stick it in their mouth to better appreciate it. As babies develop, you can watch as each of their senses is maximized for the intake of their world. Almost everything gets put in their mouths at one point or another. They touch every surface, they inhale every smell, and their eyes dart all over the place, occasionally fixing on an object and then moving on to another. Things do not have names because they don't need to; this thing is warm, that thing is wet, that other thing is slimy. A baby's world is a constant swirl of sensations, which, over time, helps them relate to their environment in increasingly meaningful ways.

This full and complete use of our senses to relate to our world is our birthright. Yet somewhere along the way, we lose the full impact of this experience and replace it with words that are shortcuts to what we are relating to but, at the same time, distance us from that experience. When we see a tree (after learning its name from our doting parents), we happily note that we "know" what it is and move on rather than appreciating the colors, shapes, and movement to which we first connected. We do not see it as we once did—we no longer connect with it because we have a label for it.

Over time, we slowly lose the full use of our senses, and we replace those sensations with intellectualizations. We are told to "grow up" and hold our emotions inside "like adults." Inexorably, we rely more and more on our mental understanding of what is going on rather than trusting what we feel. In fact, most of us are taught not to trust what we feel because it is inherently capricious and unreliable. And so our data-based brains begin to dominate over our perceptions.

Alas, our brains are easily fooled or misled. Advertising is built upon that principle: you can convince people to buy things they neither want nor need if you make it seductive enough. People can mislead us with charismatic words, but if we listen to all of the information taken in by our senses, those words will not ring "true."

Let's take a brief introductory look into how our senses are designed to process information.

Our nervous systems are designed to be affected by sound in many ways. The first sound a fetus hears is that of its mother's heartbeat. If calm, this can be calming to the fetus; if the mother is anxious or excited, her heart rate goes up and can influence the growing infant as well. That is just the beginning.

What other sounds will a baby be exposed to: an old-fashioned lullaby, soft singing, a whispering voice, or classical music perhaps? How about loud ambient noises of the city, rap or rock music, or shouts or arguments in your household? So your sense of hearing is influenced from the beginning of life by what you are exposed to. As you might expect, the natural tendency when reacting to loud sounds (which you may define as "noise") is to begin shutting down the sense of hearing to minimize the damage and over-excitation of the nervous system that it will create.

What about light? We know that to some degree light penetrates the abdominal wall so that a fetus will began to notice light prior to birth. Once born, what kinds of visual stimuli will that infant be exposed to: colors, shapes, movements, or faces? There is so much visual stimulus to choose from.

Then there's touch. The loving touch of family as they hold the baby right from the moment of birth. The baby can watch their faces, hear their voices, and feel the first of many cuddles. Are they embracing you with full acceptance, or are they timid, or even angry or scared? These experiences set the tone for a person's future as they grow.

And then there's smell and taste. Perhaps it's the mother's nipple and fresh milk, or a warmed bottle. And there are the aromas of cooking food wafting through the air. Eventually, babies will put anything they can into their mouths to taste it, feel it, and find a way to relate to it.

These are all "primitive" sensations. They are how we related to the world into which we were born. For humans, these scenarios have been playing out for millennia.

But our senses can pick that up. Our minds may be fooled. Our senses can resonate to the energies they are designed to process and inform us with accuracy about what is happening in any given moment. So we have to return to paying attention to our senses—what we see, hear, smell, taste, and touch—because that is how we can successfully navigate the complex world in which we live. In later chapters, I will discuss the need to connect to the natural world as our primary teacher and how to do it. But for now, let's embrace the concept that it is through our feelings and sensations that we will be able to connect with each other, learn from each other, and teach each other. This is the essence of energetic diagnosis.

What I am writing about is not new. Throughout recorded history, humankind has relied on the perceptual gifts of its shamans, elders, and chieftains to guide it. While, in retrospect, we may view this as primitive (as seen through the lens of "science"), perhaps we should revisit it as basic to human perception and interaction. In ancient times, the information available to tribal elders or shamans (for example, the locations of food and shelter/comfortable places to live) was viewed as critical to survival. No matter how it was (or is now) viewed, our species survived, and here we are.

In the present day, Doppler radar and satellite imaging can forecast upcoming weather systems, so we plan our days accordingly. However, I have often been impressed with the accuracy of the weather predictions from some of my patients who tell me, based on an aching knee or the onset of a headache, that a front is moving in. At times, it seems to me that their predictions are as accurate as any local weather forecast.

How did the village elders know where to winter? Where to hunt? How did the medicine men know which plants to use to treat which medical conditions? Communication with the natural world was a skill or gift that was highly honored and respected. The youngsters with a particular talent were sought after and carefully instructed to keep the knowledge of this communication alive. They were urged to practice these gifts and to pass along their knowledge to future generations.

My point is simple: learning to commune with the natural world and to learn from it was essential for human survival. We have biochemically and genetically evolved to be good at this. But, with the advances of science, these perceptions have fallen into disuse, and perhaps this is not to our benefit. It is my hope that we can delve into this subject with the intention to rediscover what is innate to us so that we can use these perceptions in the service of improving healing and communication.

How about a couple more examples? Dogs can be trained to detect the early presence of cancer. It is well known that a dog's sense of smell is infinitely more acute than a human's, but this is pretty impressive. To a lesser extent, sometimes our illnesses can alter our own perceptions to allow us to cope better. Many of my patients who develop mold toxicity find that the part of their brain referred to as the limbic system becomes far more responsive and reactive to smell, light, sound, touch, and chemicals in their environment. This means that quite a few of them can smell the presence of mold at concentrations that the folks around them cannot. Unsought, this is still a protective result of the healing process, which will allow them to avoid toxic exposures as they seek complete healing.

Having said all of this, I want to acknowledge that it may be presumptuous for me to write this book. It may be presumptuous for anyone to write such a book. I mean, given the subject at hand, how much of an expert am I—and compared to whom, exactly? But since I have already written several books, I am going to forge ahead anyway.

This book is about our abilities to perceive energies, learn from those energies, and direct them in the service of diagnosis and healing. Let me say from the outset that I am admittedly not, by any means, the most sensitive person you will encounter. I have lots of friends and colleagues who have far more profound gifts than I do.

But really, that is the point—the whole point. Why *not* me as the spokesperson for this subject, especially since I do not possess the most profound gifts? I am pretty good at experiencing some of the energies I will be discussing, and what I am trying to emphasize here is that we all have some of these gifts. If we own them, we can refine them and get better at using them. So who better to write this book than someone who is only average at this process, to convince a larger audience that this information is important and useful?

So anyone—everyone—can have energetic perception in one form or another. In fact, you already do, whether you are aware of it or not. What I hope to accomplish with this book is to start a dialogue about energetic perception so that we can share those perceptions openly and honestly and stop beating around the bush or hiding.

Unless I was going to get didactic (which would be both boring and off-target), this book is intentionally a personal story. It includes not only my story, but also the stories of several wonderful healing professionals who describe certain energies and how they interface with those energies. It is my belief that the more personal and real we get, the more you, the reader, will be able to relate to it and come aboard for the journey. Bring your own experiences and share them.

Please join me on this journey of exploration. I will introduce the material in three parts. In Part I, I share with you how I began to understand these processes. Hopefully, many of you will have had similar experiences and will not only be able to relate to them, but also realize that you too can use that information for the better. Part II digs into a number of devices and techniques that can help us perceive a variety of energies and how we can use these tools to make diagnoses and enhance treatments. I am joined by some wonderful experts who share what they have learned both professionally and personally. Finally, in Part III, we turn to the natural world, which is the source of some of the deepest perceptions available to us, and explore the experiences of several experts.

This should be fun. Come on in, the water's fine! We've been wading into it for centuries.

DISCLAIMERS

First, let me emphasize that I have no financial ties to any company, product, supplement, test, laboratory, or website mentioned in this book. If I refer to a specific product or test, it means that I have used that product or test with a great many patients and have come to appreciate how well it works. I hope that makes all such recommendations as transparent as I can make them.

Though I have made every effort to ensure the accuracy of the information presented herein, I am not engaged in providing professional advice or other services to the individual reader. The material contained in this book is not intended to be, and cannot be taken as, a substitute for the advice and counsel of one's physician and/or other healthcare providers. I shall not be liable for any loss, injury, or damage allegedly arising from any information or suggestion in this book.

Throughout this book, with a few exceptions that are clearly noted, the names of patients have been changed; all of them have consented to having their case histories presented herein. My guest authors and I have done so to protect their privacy, but we have taken care to present their medical information as accurately as possible.

PART I
The Perception of Energy and Its Value in the Diagnosis and Treatment of Illness

In the first part of this book, we are going to delve into the different types of perceptions that enable us to sense information on deeper levels—often referred to as *intuition*. I will share some personal stories that helped shape this realization, and also share some of my own perceptual gifts. It is my hope that you will relate to many of these stories and realize that you have had many of your own such experiences. Many of my patients, friends, and acquaintances have responded well to hearing these stories, and it frees them up to talk about their own stories.

For many, bringing up these experiences was too scary because of their fears about how their stories would be received. So I am opening up this whole subject for discussion. It is time that we were far more open to sharing our perceptions of the world. When we do, I know we will find that most of us have had unusual experiences.

Finally, we will discover that not only is it all right to share our perceptions, but they will be validated, too. Perhaps more important, when we get this validation, we can then allow ourselves to explore our own personal gifts, which will enable us to relate to one another on a deeper level and relate to the natural world in a way that will increase our innate sense of awe, wonderment, and joy at being part of it.

From a medical perspective, I believe that practitioners already utilize these gifts on a daily basis to make diagnoses and inform treatment, but again are reluctant to talk about it for fear of how it will look to others. However, if I can help to open up this topic for honest discussion, I believe we will become better physicians (and better people) by owning and nurturing our gifts.

So, in the first three chapters, I will share with you my own gifts and some of the life-changing events that altered my perception of the world. This will help you to better understand where I am coming from.

In Chapter 4, I explain how energies are perceived and defined in this process. Chapter 5 goes into the process of perception in more detail. This includes how a patient's perception of their own energies can help them function better. It also includes an important discussion of the difference between intuitive perception and instinctual perception, which is key to understanding which perceptions will provide us the deepest information that we can access. Then I talk about the energetic connections between humans and all other life forms, which are referred to as "energy cords."

Chapter 6 broaches the important topic of the reality of toxic and evil energies, because recognizing those energies will enable us all to protect ourselves from possible harm and be safer. In this, I am honored to have Judy Tsafrir, MD, an integrative psychiatrist, contribute her thoughts on this subject.

CHAPTER 1:
It's Time for a Change

(At Least, I Hope It Is)

The simplistic idea that we can find a single cause for a chronic, complex problem and successfully treat it is not working. How many patients have been told, based on repeated tests of blood counts and metabolic profiles (basic to the practice of medicine, currently), that they are "in the normal range," suggesting that the symptoms of their suffering cannot be verified by this outmoded approach? Far too many.

Help is on the way but is not being embraced by medical science as it should. Robert Naviaux, MD, has proposed and expanded his Cell Danger Response (CDR) model as a way for medicine to wrap its collective mind around how to understand complexity in the context of a consistent cellular response. He has developed unique blood testing using the relatively new science of metabolomics (the study of small molecules) to measure over 600 metabolites (the molecules in question) in a patient's blood with a single draw, which ultimately may help us to get a handle on different kinds of complexities within chronic illness.

Dale Bredesen, MD, is a neurologist who has put together a new understanding of Alzheimer's disease as a result of generalized inflammation, and he has demonstrated that by investigating thirty-six specific areas, we can find and successfully treat many cases of Alzheimer's. Richard Horowitz, MD, an expert on Lyme disease, has written extensively about how to evaluate a multitude of medical imbalances that contribute to the illness of Lyme and its coinfections. And I myself have written about how to investigate the many contributing factors that create chronic fatigue syndrome, fibromyalgia, Lyme disease, and mold toxicity.

What we are all describing is how to approach *complexity*—what happens when a patient is sick but doesn't exhibit medically accepted symptoms. The easy answers have evaded us, and millions of patients in the United States alone are suffering from illnesses that are going undiagnosed and untreated. So now we must learn how to dig deeper, to embrace complexity, so that we can understand how to help these unfortunate individuals.

Central to this understanding is diagnosis. It seems obvious, but bears repeating, that without a clear diagnosis, we really can't provide an effective treatment. This is not something many physicians are taught in medical school, and most of the pioneers in this field have had to learn how to do this the hard way—by trial and error.

Doing this properly requires the willingness and ability to hold multiple physiological, emotional, spiritual, and energetic imbalances in mind simultaneously and to prioritize treatments based on a patient's needs. As Dr. Naviaux has shown so clearly in several landmark medical papers, if you attempt to heal mitochondria before they are ready to accept treatment, your patient will not be able to move forward in healing. They will stay stuck. Using his model, first published in the journal *Mitochondrion* in 2013 as "Metabolic Features of the Cell Danger Response" and expanded upon in 2018, again published in the journal *Mitochondrion*, "Metabolic Features and Regulation of the Healing Cycle," we need to begin to ask the question: where, exactly, is the patient mired in the healing cycle, and what precisely do we need to do to move them forward? This is a most difficult question, but finally it is being asked, and we are beginning to find answers.

I would like to change the focus to looking for help in how to wade through the muddy waters of complexity by turning to a human capacity that has not received enough attention: intuition. Medicine has emphasized the data-based approach to diagnosis to the exclusion of everything else. If something has not been proven beyond a shadow of a doubt (which, it turns out, is very difficult to do in any laboratory), medicine casts a wary eye on it. The current terminology in conventional medicine refers to it as "evidence-based medicine."

Evidence-based medicine sounds wonderful and implies that all of our medical decisions will be based solely on intricate and detailed analyses of medical research. If it was possible for us to have access to this kind of information, I would be a proponent of this approach to the practice of medicine. Alas, it is not really as advertised.

As a physician who has published papers in peer-reviewed journals, I know how difficult it is to do good research. It is tricky, indeed, to set up an experiment with such precision that one can truly get clear and incontrovertible results. There are few papers in the medical literature than cannot be questioned based on close scrutiny of the experimental design. Given that human beings are involved in carrying out these experiments, being human, they often do not fully comply with instructions. If one delves deeply into any specific paper, there are flaws. Some of these flaws are minor, and some are major. The basic premise of evidence-based medicine is to combine all of the research done on a particular subject and then subject this mega-data to statistical interpretation. What this often means is that many flawed research papers are combined, with the concept that despite the flaws, if you crunch enough data, it will be meaningful. My view is that it is scientifically incorrect to assume that if you do this, you will get meaningful results. There is an adage: "Garbage in, garbage out." Yet this is what we have turned to in order to reassure the public that we are using only the finest standards of science to provide medical care. A number of medical writers have addressed this issue, and I encourage any reader who wants to learn more to read Dr. Ty Vincent's book, *Thinking Outside the Pill Box,* which covers this topic in more detail.

It turns out that sorting through reams of laboratory tests and complicated data is very difficult. While the current generation is convinced that computers will be able to handle this task, I am not. Computers can sort through lots of information, but they cannot hear the intonation of a patient's voice, or watch them fidget in their chair, or pause, or see their eyebrows go up as they describe their symptoms. I believe it takes another human being to become sensitive enough to those cues that they easily sort through this information to understand what is most important. This would be described as an emotion-based activity and, at this time, there is little place in medicine for it. But there should be.

It is time for us to embrace our full capacities as human beings and use all of the tools given to us at birth, including our intuition, to help us understand at a deeper level what our patients are wrestling with. In the following chapters, I will share my own stories for those aspects of diagnosis that I personally utilize; some of my esteemed colleagues will also share their experiences of diagnosing patients utilizing their intuition.

I first realized intuition was important in my first year of medical school. When we began to learn the practice of the physical examination, we went to an ENT (ear, nose, and throat) clinic to look at ears. Often, this involved my using my new otoscope, looking into the ear, and trying to understand what I was looking at. As you might imagine, in that particular clinic we saw quite a few ear infections.

One of my first surprises was that my teachers (professors, residents, and interns) could not agree on what they were seeing in each ear. All that was involved in this exercise was looking into the ear with the aid of a bright light and moving your otoscope around to see as much of the eardrum and ear canal as you could—that's it. You would think that, like looking at a purple flower, everyone would agree that we were looking at a purple flower. Not so. When I realized early on that there were significant discrepancies in what we were seeing, I would draw what I saw, and then ask the intern, resident, and attending physician to draw what they saw. Rarely did these drawing agree. When examining a child with ear pain, sometimes one or more of these physicians would see a red eardrum, sometimes a retracted (pulled-back) eardrum, or an eardrum with a muffled "light reflex," which refers to a cone of light that should be reflected by a normal eardrum. Rarely did all four of us draw the same picture or see the same thing. I was flabbergasted. How could this be?

I came to realize that a physician's diagnostic opinion had a lot to do with what they "saw." What I mean is that if the physician thought the child needed antibiotics, they invariably saw a red eardrum. If they thought the child had increased pressure in the eustachian tube and the eardrum was retracted, and did not need antibiotics, that was what they saw.

It was fascinating—what a physician saw was directly related to their intuition about what they were going to use for treatment! When I attempted to share these perceptions with my teachers, they ignored me. What this experience taught me was that what guided their diagnosis and treatment was their intuition about what they thought their patient had. No one else said a single word about this phenomenon throughout my entire time in medical school.

I have observed this dynamic play out time and time again during my forty-nine years of medical practice. I have taught as an assistant director in a family practice residency program and at the University of Minnesota at Duluth School of Medicine, and worked with hundreds and hundreds of physicians over the years; still, rarely does anyone acknowledge that they are using intuition constantly in their medical practice. If you are paying attention, you will notice that the best physicians use it all the time. It is a fabulous tool for connecting with patients, helping to make diagnoses, and coming up with a treatment plan.

My hope that we can more formally open a dialogue about how important intuition is in the practice of medicine and begin to focus on it, teach it, and utilize it in the service of healing.

CHAPTER 2:
My Diagnostic Gifts

LAYING MY CARDS ON THE TABLE (and Those Are Not Tarot Cards)

Many people consider me to be an excellent diagnostician, and I hope that this reputation is deserved. I have treated thousands of patients who were extremely ill and assisted in bringing many, if not most, of them back to health.

How did I develop those skills?

Allow me to share the things I do when a new patient comes into my office, which enables me to arrive at the best diagnosis possible given the information available to me. (Please keep in mind that my practice has evolved over the years into a referral practice; most of these patients have been quite ill for many years and not improved under conventional, and sometimes unconventional, medical care. Many have been bedridden and have had a multitude of diagnostic labels assigned to them, which has not allowed them to make progress.)

To start, I greet each patient in the waiting room and accompany them to my little office. In the waiting area, I notice how well they are able to get up from the couch or chair, and I see how they walk down the hall. I am already logging mental notes about their movement and gait that will be helpful to me. My patients are not placed in a gown and asked to wait around on an uncomfortable examination table in a chilly room for ten to twenty minutes before I arrive.

Then we sit down face-to-face, and I take handwritten notes. (My computer remains behind me, and I rarely touch it during a consultation.) For the most part, I just listen to them describe what has happened to them and how they feel. I listen not just with my ears but with my whole body. With my eyes, I take in whether they fidget in their seat or settle in comfortably. I notice when certain words or descriptions make them react. I notice their breathing, their pauses, and their silences. I ask lots of questions to flush out their stories. Patients often do not know what I need to know to help them, so I push for details. If a description is vague, I need more. I need to know how their symptoms have affected them physically, emotionally, and spiritually. If these effects are not clear, I need to ask more questions. My initial evaluation is scheduled for two hours, and I often need more time than that. I encourage patients to record the session so they can review it later. (Many of my patients are cognitively impaired and need this review.)

During this entire conversation, it is my intention to listen with every fiber of my being. First and foremost, I ask: what are your expectations for our visit today? Then, when did your health begin to decline? Did anything happen to you about that time to contribute to that decline? What stresses were you under? How did this stress affect you? What followed afterward (like a domino effect)? What are your major symptoms today? Which of those symptoms affect you the most?

While asking these questions and allowing my patient to tell their story as completely as they can, I am paying attention to patterns. Does this narrative relate to others that I have heard? Do the details fit together into a pattern that makes sense—that explains what they have been experiencing—or is this story somehow incomplete? Am I missing details that would clarify their experience? What haven't they told me, or what don't I know that will help me make a diagnosis? Throughout this process, I strive to maintain a focus—a prayer, if you will—asking for divine guidance in being attuned to what I am experiencing so that I can really hear what the patient is asking for at the deepest level that they are capable of communicating that information.

Following this verbal consultation, I often sit in silence with my patient for a few moments, allowing this information to "percolate" through me so I can formulate my thoughts into a cohesive pattern that puts all of this information together. To make my patient more comfortable with my silence, I first reassure them that I just need to think for a few moments to sort through everything they have told me. Virtually every patient responds to this request with, "Oh, please, take all the time you need to think it through." Then I perform a physical examination to be sure I am not missing anything or to confirm some findings that are likely to be present or absent given the story I have heard. Finally, I outline for my patient, and the family and friends who accompany them, how I can make sense of this information, what I think needs to be treated, and in what order.

At the end of our session, I provide handwritten instructions and a plan and schedule a follow-up visit.

So what makes my patient examinations different from what other physicians are doing, besides some flowery phrases and lofty ideals? Nothing. I do, however, have a few gifts that allow me to be an active participant in this process. These gifts enable me to sort through all of the complicated information and tease out what is important from what may not be.

THE GIFT OF KNOWING
(or, as I Call It, Claircognizance)

Over my forty-nine years of medical practice, I have come to realize that I am absorbing information in ways that are generally not discussed. I did not learn this approach in medical school. My patients taught me how to do it, often unwittingly, but not without my eventual gratitude.

My primary gift, which it took me a while to understand, is the gift of "knowing." What this means, simply, is that sometimes in sitting with a patient, I just know information about them without them saying anything.

The first time this happened was relatively dramatic. I was several years out of medical training, and I had been studying hypnosis and emotional release therapy in the form of Reichian therapy. I was working as a family physician in a small town in northern California and also helping in the local hospital's ER and maternity ward delivering babies. Through these hospital tours, I had become known to other local physicians as having an ability and interest in applying alternative medicine to difficult problems. A gynecologist in the area wound up referring a young woman to me who had recurrent ovarian cysts and bouts of abdominal pain that were so frequent she was having difficulty functioning. The referring physician (here, "intuition" comes into play again) thought that somehow I could help her patient because repeat surgeries and hospitalizations were not proving effective.

Honestly, I had no idea what I could do, but I invited the young woman to my office and just listened to her story.

As she spoke, a message appeared as if typed in my field of vision. It read: "Ask her about the time she was raped." Whoa! What in the world was this message about? I had never experienced such a thing before. Could I just blurt out that horrible question? How inappropriate would that be? But she continued to relate her story, and a second "typed" message appeared across my field of vision, this time more insistent: "Ask her about the time she was raped!" Again, I resisted. This was too weird, and asking such a question would be an invasion of her privacy. I don't do things like that. I am a very respectful physician. It would not be right! She continued speaking, and a third message practically screamed at me: "Ask her about the time she was raped!"

I did not know how to respond. Torn between being rude or trusting this bizarre message, I finally gathered up my courage and, while questioning my sanity, hesitantly said: "Tell me about the time you were raped."

Her response was stunning. She broke down sobbing and slowly told me how, at age fourteen, her sister's husband had raped her one night while she was babysitting their children. As if that was not horrific enough, no one believed her. When she became pregnant, she was ostracized from the family and tossed out into the street. Now, ten years later and married, she was still hurting from this trauma, which was affecting her relationship and sexual connection with her husband.

Was this trauma the cause of her recurrent ovarian cysts? I had no idea, but I allowed this experience to evolve and worked with it in whatever way I could.

After hearing her story, I mentioned my background with hypnosis and emotional release work and explained that if a patient could relive an old trauma and release the emotions they had been holding for many years, sometimes healing could take place. I asked if I could use hypnosis to regress her to that event so she could release the emotional pain that was stored in her body, presumably in her pelvic area. She gave her permission, and without difficulty she summoned a clear memory/experience of that event. With my support, she was able to release the intense anxiety, fear, sadness, and grief from that experience over several sessions. Her health improved immediately, as did her marriage. Her ovarian cysts never recurred.

I wasn't sure how to make sense of that intense experience, but several features seemed important at the time. First, after receiving the same "typed" message three times and in an increasingly adamant way, I eventually took a leap of faith and trusted that message; I could utilize it to ask a question that I would otherwise be reticent to ask. I did not know its source, but since it led to a therapeutic breakthrough, it seemed remarkably helpful. Second, I trusted that I had the tools to use that information to bring about healing for this troubled young woman.

Given the unique nature of this event, I find it difficult to explain why I decided to respect the "message" that I was receiving. Perhaps others, in the same situation, would not. This is where "faith" enters the picture. All I can relate is that despite how inappropriate the question was, I knew on some level that in the end, asking it would be helpful to my patient. And, with a great deal of trepidation, I asked the question, knowing that I was risking a terrible outcome if I was wrong. Hence this was a life-changing experience for both me and this young woman in my care.

Several months later, another of my patients was admitted to the local hospital with a wide array of symptoms, and the ER doctor did not know what was wrong. When I arrived at the patient's bedside, another typed message came across my visual field: "He has viral meningitis." This was a bit surprising to me because he did not have a headache, a stiff neck, or a fever, and the rest of his laboratory work was negative; we had no answer for what was making him so ill. So again, I took a chance and acted on this "information" I had been given; we wound up doing a spinal tap to look at his spinal fluid. If I had been wrong, I could have harmed the patient, and certainly I had no clear indication that this diagnosis was medically indicated. But, as it turned out, the spinal tap was clearly positive. He did, indeed, have an unusual presentation of spinal meningitis, and we were able to successfully treat it.

Some of my colleagues were amazed at this diagnostic "coup," but I was more amazed that I had trusted this information and that, once again, the outcome was a good one.

Over the next few years, I would occasionally get those typed messages, and they were never wrong. Eventually, they stopped coming, but I was now being given that information directly so I became aware that I "knew" something without having any idea of how. The transition from typed messages that came across my visual field to a direct perception of "knowing" that information occurred so gradually that I was unaware of it for some time. When this information came to me, it was associated with a "feeling" that it was not "me" who knew it, so I knew I could rely on this sensed information as accurate and different from my usual thought processes.

It still does not happen with every patient I encounter, but this "knowing" has become a part of my diagnostic process. If I sit still and listen carefully, it often comes to me. It is always worth listening to.

I have no idea how this happens; it just does. This gift is what I consider to be my deepest intuition; I have learned not to question it, but to use it in the service of healing. As you might imagine, it comes in quite handy when dealing with complicated patients. While my left brain, where analytical thinking is generated, is quite well trained and very helpful, combining it with my emotionally intelligent right brain and what we call "intuition" definitely helps. It turns out to be an excellent combination.

It is important to understand that with each gift comes a liability. To maximize the gift, you have to fully comprehend the liability so that it does not set you back. While you might imagine that "knowing" would be cool, I can assure you that you will not always want to know the information you are gaining access to. This information may include becoming aware of behaviors and attitudes that the patient would much rather you not know. When this applies to friends and acquaintances, it is imperative that you do not share what you are picking up or you will run the risk of offending that person, sometimes irreparably.

To give you an example, early in my medical career I realized that I could "see" the "inner light" or potential that others possessed. Since I had no idea that everyone couldn't do this, I became upset when my friends were not maximizing their potential. Being rather naïve, when I pushed them to be their best selves, they would often get mad at me for holding them to an ideal that *I* could see, but they were not yet ready to embrace. In fact, I lost my best friend when I made just such an accusation one day, and he turned his back on me for asking him for something he felt he was not ready for. I did not understand it then, but I do now. Everyone needs to be allowed the time and respect to shape their own future and their own destiny. No one needs my input on that. So, if you have been granted this gift, please use it wisely. Pushing someone to embrace information that they do not feel ready to process will only push them away and make them more defensive.

THE GIFT OF FEELING
(aka Clairsentience)

Often referred to as "empathy," clairsentience describes the ability to *feel* what someone else is feeling—not merely to understand it, but to feel it. While this is not my strongest gift, it has slowly evolved over the years in a way that is especially helpful to me for making diagnoses.

The first time this gift was brought to my attention, I was treating a patient by delving deep into her emotional past. A medical student was shadowing me to learn about my style of practicing; all of a sudden, I felt a sharp pain in my chest. It is hard for me to explain, but the pain did not feel like it belonged to me. We all have our own unique ways of perceiving, and this wasn't in alignment with my typical perceptions. I assumed that the pain was coming from the patient I was treating, but when I asked her if she was experiencing chest pain, to my surprise she responded that she was not. I wasn't sure what to make of that, but we completed our therapy session and she left the room. It was then that the medical student confessed that she was feeling chest pain. The emotional events being processed by my patient had touched my student too close to home. Ultimately, this led to a therapeutic breakthrough for my student. It also helped me to understand that I needed to honor what I was feeling and explore where that feeling was coming from to be of optimal service.

While empathy allows those with this gift to connect at a deep level with those around them (which is a good thing), those with the gift of feeling often do not realize that they need to explore whose feelings they are perceiving. Many assume that everything they feel comes from within themselves and become quite confused. It is common for those with this gift to enter a crowded room feeling comfortable and soon become depressed, sad, or morose for no reason. They often do not realize that they are picking up the feelings of someone else in the room, and they are often moved to leave without understanding why. They may even feel poorly for hours or days afterward, with no clear reasons.

It is helpful for those with this gift to learn to ask themselves, "Whose feelings are these?" repeatedly, until they begin to automatically clarify this origin for themselves on a regular basis. The gift of feeling allows an individual to perceive that a particular feeling is not "theirs" because it does not *feel* like theirs, and the sooner they can let it go, the less likely they are to be disturbed by it.

A variation on this theme is important to the subject of energetic diagnosis. Taking myself as an example, I have treated so many patients with chronic fatigue, fibromyalgia, Lyme disease, and mold toxicity that over time, I can "feel" how those illnesses have impacted the energy of my patient. Patients with mold toxicity "feel" different than those with Lyme disease or coinfections. I have come to trust these feelings implicitly. When I am attempting to sort through a complicated patient history, it is extremely helpful to be able to home in on certain possibilities with this perception. If I combine my gift of knowing with this perception, it is of great help in diagnostic clarity. Please understand that some patients do not radiate this clarity of energy, and occasionally I am baffled by what I am experiencing. This means that I need to spend more time with this patient, and gaining the clarity we need to move forward may require additional visits. I would like to emphasize that a clear diagnosis is critical to helping every patient. Without that clarity, we are simply "shooting in the dark," which is not a good strategy for providing medical care.

While this description may seem a bit too far "out there," I would like you to know that a number of healing traditions utilize these perceptions and hone them as a part of their educational curriculum. Most notably, osteopathic medicine has for generations trained those who are specializing in manual/manipulational medicine to perceive what a wide variety of biochemical perturbations feel like. (Low blood sugar, low magnesium, and high blood pressure are examples.) When my colleague Jeffrey Greenfield, DO, realized that he could feel the vibrations of Lyme disease and mold toxicity (to help him with both diagnosis and treatment), he created a course through which he has trained dozens of physicians to feel these illnesses directly.

While some people may be skeptical of everything I am describing here, one of my major motivations in writing about this perception is that I am convinced that many physicians already have these experiences but are reluctant to talk about them for fear of what others might think. As for me, I have passed the age that I care about that and hope that these descriptions will stimulate a more honest and open dialogue about these experiences so that medicine can embrace this is a subject worthy of study and training.

THE GIFT OF SEEING

There are many gifts of seeing, many of them named as clairvoyance or given labels like precognition, premonition, prophecy, aura reading, telepathy, and second sight. I will talk more about this in later chapters, but here I want to focus on my own perception so you can understand the background with which I frame this information. All of these abilities, often referred to as psychic abilities, are separate, and individuals vary quite a bit in terms of which gifts they are best suited to work with. For example, I do not see auras. I am, however, somewhat telepathic, especially with my wife. She and I often recognize that we are having the same thought or plan, and it is often unclear which of us came up with it first. I suspect that this began to occur early in our relationship, but it took a while for both of us to recognize that it was happening. At this stage in our thirty-year relationship, we joke about not knowing which of us had the thought first.

I want to come back to something I mentioned earlier in this chapter: I realized early on (in my twenties) that I could see what I call the "inner light" inside another human being. This is not an aura perception, but a sense of that individual's energy, or life force, or spark of vitality, and it gives me a feeling about what they may be capable of becoming. As noted previously, this ability got me into quite a bit of trouble until I learned not to say anything about what I was perceiving. I lost several close friends until I began to grasp what was going on. After all, I assumed that if I could perceive their potential, surely so could they! I can assure you that this is not the case. However, after many years of making and following observations, I realized that this could be very useful in deciding which patients I wished to follow closely and stick with—no matter how slow their progress—and which ones I needed to dismiss so they could find someone better suited to their needs. Over decades, I have discovered that when I can see a patient's inner light and I continue to help them on the path to healing, they will get there eventually, even if it takes five to ten years. If I did not see that light but kept working with them anyway in the mistaken belief that somehow we would find their answer, they did not recover under my care. It took me years of not helping those patients to realize that it was better for both my patients and me to honor that perception and encourage them to find another physician who could perhaps be more helpful for them. If I cannot help a patient, it is important not to blame anyone for that lack of progress but to acknowledge it early on and let that patient move on.

THE GIFT OF PERCEIVING MENTAL IMAGES

There probably is a name for this gift, but I am not aware of it. What I am aware of is that at times, I can see the pictures that someone in my presence is creating in their mind as they talk about something.

My children have found this ability very disturbing. When they were younger and tried to lie to me, I could see the images in their minds. When those images did not match the words coming out of their mouths, I knew I was hearing a story. As they became aware of this, even if they did not know what was happening, they became less and less willing to lie to me. I recall my daughter, at age eight or nine, yelling at me one day, "You cannot possibly know that!" What the children did not know, and I never told them (although the cat is now officially out of the bag), is that I cannot always see these pictures; it is not constant like all of the other perceptions I have talked about. But I could do it often enough to make them wary of making things up.

This gift can be helpful to me when working with patients because if a patient's verbal story does not jibe with the mental pictures I am seeing, I know that what they are telling me is what they want me to think, even if it is not true. I never share these perceptions with my patients—accusing them of lying or distorting the truth would get us nowhere fast—but I file them away for possible future use.

MOVING FORWARD

I believe that every human being has multiple gifts like the ones I have. I believe that exploring these gifts, especially those that are the most innate to each individual, will enhance our ability to communicate with one another at deeper, more profound levels and make the possibilities of our lives even more exciting and marvelous. By maximizing our potential for seeing the world as the energetic wonder that it is, it can only get better if we learn to use these gifts with respect and care. In medicine, it is time for us to discuss this openly and honestly and give our perceptions room to flourish.

CHAPTER 3:
Opening Oneself Up to Perceptual Shifts: Life-Changing Experiences

I believe that most of us have experienced unusual "coincidences." Whether or not we allow those experiences to shape us, inform us, or affect us determines in large part how we view the world we live in. You can consider these experiences to be divinely inspired, magical, amazing, or just random coincidences; that is up to you.

In this book, I share several of my own experiences because they have had a lot to do with shaping my view of the universe I inhabit and my awareness of it. These stories might help you to understand how I arrived at the worldview that underlies this book. I believe that most of you who are reading this book have had similar, or even more profound, experiences. Some of you came away with a deep feeling of awe about the world that surrounds us. Others, perhaps more skeptical or even jaded, were less impressed. It is not the experience you have as much as how you come to view it.

So here are three of my formative stories.

THE NUTCRACKER:
THE BIRD, NOT THE BALLET

In the late 1970s, I went on a backpacking trip through Yosemite in late September with my dear, now-departed friend Stan Weisenberg. Stan was an exceptional chiropractor and my traveling buddy for many years. On this particular trip, Stan wanted to learn how to use a compass and an altimeter to guide us through uncharted territory—an interesting metaphor, as you will see. Since I had learned to use these devices in my Boy Scout training, I felt confident that I could provide backup if needed, and we planned our jaunt through the wilderness.

With our packs loaded up, we set off from one of the trails of southern Yosemite to find our way to Beaver Lake, where we planned to spend the night. On the maps we carried, it appeared that if we got to one specific area, we could hike the rim of a canyon and get to a spot that descended to the lake.

About a mile into our trip, we took off across the terrain on no specific trail, using only our compass, altimeter, and map to guide us. After about an hour of hiking, it became apparent that we had no idea where we were, and our compass and altimeter were no longer working. By that I mean that within very short distances, the altimeter would read either 7,000 feet or 1,500 feet, and it was clear that those readings were now useless. Similarly, the compass readings shifted dramatically from moment to moment.

We were out in the middle of nowhere and had no idea where exactly we were or how to go forward or backward. We took off our packs, sat down in the forest, and tried to figure out what to do. Stymied, we just could not decide on our next step.

When Stan and I were at our most desperate, a Clark's nutcracker popped up on a branch ahead of us and chattered away with its screeching call. (For those of you who are not birders, as I was, it looks somewhat similar to a jay with black wings and white sides.) Then it hopped onto a branch several yards down the trail and seemed to wait. I cannot explain it, but it seemed to be communicating with me. It flew back to its original branch and then popped back again.

Out of ideas, I told Stan, "I'm going to follow the bird." Appalled, Stan suggested I might be out of my mind. I agreed that I might, but I put my pack back on and said, "Do you have a better idea?" So we followed the bird, who methodically flew ahead of us for several miles, going from branch to branch. Then, at the edge of a precipice, the nutcracker suddenly flew between two boulders and was gone.

Still unsure of what to do, I implored Stan to follow the route the bird had begun to take through the rocks. To my surprise, we found a faint but definite trail that snaked its way through the boulders on the way down a steep 300-foot embankment, eventually winding up at the base of the cliff and a lake in the visible distance. We checked the map and saw that we had actually arrived at Beaver Lake.

I cannot describe the relief Stan and I felt when we arrived at our intended destination. We looked up at the cliff above us, at what we had originally thought might be a trail to get down to the lake, and realized it did not exist. There is no way we could have achieved that goal on our own. Although it is a cliché: the hair on the backs of our necks began to tingle and stand right up. We knew we had experienced something amazing. A bird had led us through the wilderness!

In retrospect, we had been led effortlessly, seamlessly, along the only route we could have taken, by trusting the idea (which even to me seemed crazy at the time) that a wild creature could save us. It is difficult to explain my decision to trust the nutcracker. Perhaps, in the way that it looked at me directly and flew from its nearby branch to one a bit farther away and back again, it seemed to be beckoning to me. Before I decided to follow it, I did question whether that was even possible. When we reached our destination, I knew that this experience had been transformative. It put an exclamation point on my generally held (but unproven) opinion that the natural world is nurturing to those who hold it in high esteem and that you can trust it with your life. I had always loved the natural world, but now that love was coupled with a deep-seated belief that it loved me back.

As an interesting counterpoint to this experience, I would like to refer you to a couple of recent books by the ornithologist Jennifer Ackerman, *The Genius of Birds* and *The Bird Way: A New Look at How Birds Talk, Work, Play, Parent and Think*, published in 2016 and 2020, respectively. In *The Genius of Birds*, Ackerman does a masterful job of reviewing the scientific research, which shows that birds are far more intelligent than we realized. Of particular interest is that jays (a family to which the Clark's nutcracker belongs) are among the most intelligent bird species. Her most recent book details how birds communicate very clearly not only with other birds but with humans as well.

AN ALMOST BIBLICAL STORY _____

When my eldest son, Jules, was just four years old, he had a severe episode of croup. Croup is a typically viral illness that occurs during winter, in which the epiglottis, a flap of tissue at the base of the throat, swells up and interferes with breathing. Some children are predisposed to this illness, as Jules was. He had had mild episodes of croup every year.

One cold December night, when Jules was suffering from his yearly episode, he came into our bedroom and was having obvious difficulty breathing. I put him in a hot shower room and then took him outside in the frigid Duluth weather (switching from hot to cold environments often breaks an attack), but nothing I did seemed to help. Jules's breathing became more and more labored. Doctor Neil shares hats with Father Neil, and Father Neil was freaking out.

I prepared to take Jules to the emergency room, but in case his breathing shut down before we could get there, I put a knife in my pocket and steeled myself for the possibility that I might need to use it. If his breathing stopped completely, I would need to make a slit in his throat to open up his breathing below the obstruction. I knew how to do this, but I'd never had any occasion to. Terrified that this drastic step might become necessary, I put Jules in the car and got ready to go.

As often happens with this illness, all of sudden Jules began to breathe more normally, and the crisis passed. He was okay and then healed quickly afterward. But I was not okay. Although I had prepared myself for the worst, when I knew that Jules was safe, I began to shake intensely and cry. I continued to cry, actually sob, not only that night, but off and on for the next six or seven weeks. The floodgates had opened, and I could not close them.

Many of those around me—my family, my friends, and my patients—did not know how to relate to sobbing Neil. It was a strange phenomenon as well. While I was, indeed, sobbing much of the day, it did not feel "bad," just odd. It felt, on an intuitive level, like something that I needed to allow myself to go through. The reality that I was prepared to use a knife to open my son's trachea to allow him to breathe hit me to my core, and it triggered some kind of healing release; it was something I had to experience in full. So I didn't fight it. I was a bit more tired than usual and had to cut my workday down from eight to nine hours to six or seven hours. Many of my patients were baffled by my behavior and expressed their concern as to whether or not was I alright. Even more important, they wondered whether I could responsibly focus on their care and not compromise it. I was sure that I could. And that's what I did.

Eventually, my sobbing subsided and then stopped; I became "Neil" again. But I knew that I was, somehow, changed. The crying jags did not trigger any specific event or experience that I could recall—no traumatic memories—but perhaps a lifetime of stored emotion poured out of me, and I trusted my body enough to know that I would be better off if I just let it happen.

As I reflect on this event and acknowledge that I do not understand the specifics of what happened to me, I feel that it provided a necessary opportunity for me to open myself up to a fuller experience and appreciate the world around me. It made me more perceptive, especially of emotion in both myself and others. Since then, several of my patients have described very similar experiences, which resulted in their healing.

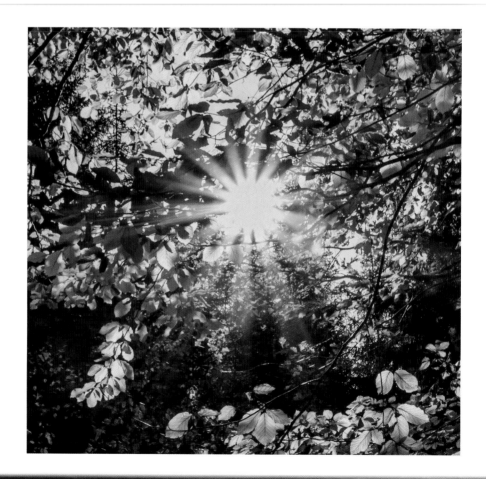

ON DEATH AND DYING _____

HOW DO YOU KNOW WHEN SOMEONE HAS TRULY DIED?

Spoiler Alert: You Don't.

In 1974, after I completed my stint with the Indian Health Service in Alaska, I set up my first medical practice in Fort Bragg, California. This consisted of working a twenty-four-hour shift in the emergency room every week: delivering babies, performing minor surgeries, and caring for hospitalized patients.

One of my patients was an elderly woman who had developed failure of almost every major organ system of her body. She had heart failure, respiratory failure, and kidney failure. To top it off, she had developed a "web" of tissue that spanned her esophagus, which allowed only a 1 mm opening through which she could swallow food or drink. What this meant was that we could hardly keep her hydrated or provide adequate nutrition within the context of a body that was failing. Despite this, she managed to continue to function, not well, but not getting worse either, for about nine months. As you might expect, it would not have taken too much strain to overload her fragile system.

One night when I was working my ER shift, my elderly patient's family brought her in gasping for breath. She had caught a cold, and that was all it took to precipitate a catastrophic result.

We stabilized her in the ER and then transferred her to our intensive care unit, where we provided oxygen and tried our best to stabilize her failing systems. She had a tube in her throat (so she could breathe), another tube in her arm for fluids, and EKG leads to monitor her heart activity. While I was attending to her, she suddenly stopped breathing. We formally called a "code," meaning that the nursing staff, respiratory therapist, and I did everything in our power to resuscitate her. Her family was not ready to let her go, and she herself had expressed that she was not ready to die yet.

But after twenty minutes of every type of resuscitation method and technique we knew of, her EKG leads showed no heart activity ("straight line"), she was not breathing without us pushing on her chest, and she had no pulse. We'd done all we could, but she was gone.

Or so we thought. As I formally pronounced her "dead" and began the process of removing all of the tubes, all of a sudden her EKG leads, which were still attached, fired up and showed a normal heart rate! This was not possible! All of the medical personnel in attendance looked at each other in awe and wonder. Then she began to breathe again (still gasping for air, but breathing in a labored way as she had been before), regained full consciousness, and asked for specific family members to approach her because she needed to share some things with them. She did this for over an hour. The nursing staff and I were unable to process what we were witnessing. She had not taken a breath in over twenty minutes, and, by everything we had ever been taught, it was not possible for a person to revive after not getting any oxygen for even five minutes. But she did. After giving cogent last-minute instructions to her family, she stopped breathing again, just as suddenly as she had "come back to life." This time, she did not recover.

To put this experience in context, having been called to the bedside for many years for hospital patients who had stopped breathing and whose hearts had stopped beating, I had agonized about the correct length of time to continue to attempt resuscitation. I am not alone in that dilemma. This is the one time in medical practice when we literally have to "play God." The decision to continue efforts of resuscitation lies with the physician alone. How can we know when a patient has died with any precision? Should we keep going? For how long? What state of health will this patient be in if we succeed? Will this prolonged absence of oxygen and blood have damaged their brain or other organs?

I will be eternally grateful to this woman for answering this question. She let me know, in no uncertain terms, that I did not decide. She did.

Despite the fact that not having a heartbeat or breath for twenty minutes supposedly makes it impossible to survive, she returned to her previous state of health as if nothing had happened. She was lucid, completed the communications with her family that were so important to her, and then really did die.

I hope I can share with you how profoundly this experience changed my view of the responsibilities I have for those who are close to dying. I cannot speak for other physicians, but the thought that "I" decided whether someone lived or died, and when, was a huge weight upon me. Now, I realized that this decision was never mine to make. If someone was able to take the efforts at resuscitation we were providing and use them to recover, they would survive. If they were ready for death, or if our efforts were not sufficient, so be it. I know that many of you have your own beliefs about God and the divine, but to me, this was absolute proof that God and the patient, together, decided.

I can generalize from this experience to a larger belief of mine, that the outcome of any effort at healing I attempt to provide again is dependent on my patient and God, not me. This takes a huge burden from my shoulders and allows me to practice medicine. If I felt personally responsible for every decision and choice my patients made, good or bad, I am not sure I could live with that burden. Fortunately, I don't have to. That's up to God. I just work here. Yes, I always do my best, and sometimes my best is not enough. But I don't decide that. Knowing, to the depth of my being, that there is a bigger plan out there, one that I am rarely privy to, allows me to keep doing my best and hoping for the best every day. And although this story is not directly about intuition, it is the clearest experience I have had about the presence of a higher power that ultimately has far more influence on the outcomes of medical interventions than I do.

While there are many more stories to recount (and there will be more to read from my contributing authors and myself), these three have had a profound effect on my perspective of the natural world, the value of emotion and emotional release in healing, and my role in providing healthcare. I hope that this background will help you to understand what I bring to the table when we discuss the gifts of perception and healing that are at the core of this book.

CHAPTER 4:
What Is Energy, and How Can It Be Perceived?

Let me begin by trying to get some kind of definition of energy out of the way. It is a task at which I may not succeed. As science writer Cathal O'Connell notes, energy is "one of the most basic concepts in physics but one of the hardest to define."

One way to attempt a definition is to use the discipline of physics, which tells us that energy is the capacity to do work. I am not sure how useful that is in the context of this book. If we look at Einstein's famous equation $E = mc^2$, what does that mean? I have little grasp of the concept of the c, the speed of light, and attempting to square that number leaves me baffled. The idea of multiplying those already mind-bending numbers by m, or mass, leaves me pretty much nowhere. At the risk of appearing less than erudite, I confess that I cannot fully place this equation into any context that is meaningful to me, so I will abandon any effort to use those definitions offered by physics to help us understand how to conceptualize energy. I do not see how a long discussion of whether energy is kinetic or potential would bring us any closer to understanding how we can experience it and use it in the service of healing.

I would rather discuss energy from the perspective of how we perceive it, which I believe is intuitive and obvious for most people. We perceive energy in many ways:

- We can see it with our eyes as light or motion. For example, some painters, such as Monet, are noted for their ability to detect tiny differences in color or light and convey them on canvas.

- We can feel it with our bodies and hands as motion or temperature changes (heat or cold). Those with sensitive hands make exceptional masseuses or healers.

- We can hear it in the changes of sound waves in the form of tone, pitch, loudness or softness, or musicality. Those who have an ear for sound can compose beautiful symphonies by combining notes.

- We may be able to smell it in the form of odors or scents. Perfumers use their sensitive noses to combine scents in pleasing ways.

- We may be able to taste it as well. Gourmet chefs and wine tasters are described as having an unusually refined palate. They are sensitive to and can detect flavors and aromas that others cannot.

My point is simply that the experience of energy is personal and individual. We are all biochemically and genetically different, and we are neurologically wired to experience these stimuli in our own unique ways. Each of us has our own particular *gifts* for perception, or perhaps has our own particular preferences for perception.

At the root of this discussion is the ability to perceive some form of energy and utilize this perception in the service of creativity. This is not rocket science. Everyone has some of these gifts, in various combinations, and everyone has had some experience with utilizing these perceptions in daily life.

THE BASICS OF PERCEPTUAL PREFERENCES

For many years, educators have found it useful to talk about perceptual learning preferences. It should come as no surprise that our learning preferences are directly related to our perceptual gifts. For example, a person who is auditory would be much more likely to respond to auditory stimuli. Our perceptions are broken down into three basic categories:

AUDITORY   **VISUAL**   **KINESTHETIC**

Those whose have a preference for auditory learning do better at acquiring information while listening—for example, to a lecture or podcast. They may move their lips and read aloud. And in my experience at medical meetings, they also enjoy question-and-answer sessions.

Those who prefer visual perception fall into two subcategories: linguistic and spatial.

People who have a visual-linguistic learning preference like to learn through written language. They can remember what has been written down, even if they do not reread it.

Those who are visual-spatial learners may have difficulty with the written word but do well with videos, charts, and demonstrations. Many people with this preference can readily grasp concepts from watching YouTube presentations. They also have an innate sense of direction, which is reflected as an increased awareness of space and their relationship to that space.

Those who learn best using kinesthetic intake prefer touching and moving. While reading, they may underline passages, take notes on the page, or use colored pens for emphasis. After listening to several lectures, a kinesthetic learner's brain may begin to feel overwhelmed, and they may have to move around in their chair, get up and take a walk, or just take a break, or they will become antsy.

Which of these perceptions do you primarily use? I am both visual-linguistic and kinesthetic: I experience the world primarily through my eyes and my sense of touch. I am not very auditory. I can listen to a lecture over and over again, but if I don't take notes (the kinesthetic part), not much will sink in; furthermore, my notes must be handwritten, not typed. I use stars to emphasize what I think is important: one star means interesting, two stars more so, and three, even more critical. I use arrows to indicate that I should come back and review key information. Perhaps I am a dinosaur, but taking notes on a computer or tablet does not have the same effect for me. So, if you catch me at a medical meeting, I will not be sitting in front of a laptop, but will have a paper pad in front of me, writing down my reactions to what I am hearing as quickly as I can. Here is the interesting part: I rarely look at those notes again, but the simple act of writing them down helps me remember that information. My brain seems to accept the fact that the act of taking notes means that it needs to pay attention to what I am writing.

Similarly, I am not a spatial learner; I have no sense of direction whatsoever. I map out directions and study them rather than use GPS. My wife, Cheryl, meanwhile, seldom gets lost in an unfamiliar environment, using her imagination to visualize her surroundings.

In my experience, these are not merely learning preferences; over time we train our brains to respond to these stimuli. Using myself as an example, my senses of touch and sight are quite refined. Drawn to these stimuli, I have studied osteopathic manipulation and massage techniques for many years and have gained some skill with my hands in the process. I read voraciously and enjoy it. On the other hand, my appreciation of sound is much less. I now require hearing aids, and I do not enjoy listening to music because my interaction with auditory stimuli has declined. I prefer quiet.

Please keep in mind that all of us have some ability to learn from and appreciate auditory, visual, and kinesthetic information. It is just that we are all different biochemically, neurologically, and genetically, and we all have our own unique preferences. There is no right or wrong or good or bad preference; it is just how we are wired. What matters is that the better we can appreciate our personal preferences or gifts, the more comfortably we can select the living and learning environments in which we place ourselves and, by doing so, optimize our experience.

MORE SOPHISTICATED PERCEPTIONS

The perceptions I am going to get into next comprise the essence of this book. These more sophisticated perceptions have been ascribed to virtually every leader from every spiritual tradition. I want to make sure that we do not trivialize these individuals by dismissing them as "psychic" or having "ESP." Millions of people accept that Jesus turned water into wine and provided enough loaves and fishes for a gathered assembly. Similarly, millions accept that Moses parted the Red Sea, or that the Buddha could look into the heart of an individual and realize that that person had the potential to injure countless, blameless countrymen. While those who are more scientifically oriented search for more "reasonable" explanations for these recorded events, even those who question the veracity of these legends will admit that at least some tiny part of them wonders if the legends might be true—and perhaps even hopes that they are.

Most of us have had at least a few experiences that logic alone cannot explain. The more of these experiences we have, the more willing we may be to explore these perceptions further. It is also true that some people are frightened by these events and refuse to accept them, declining to allow any further hint of such experiences into their consciousness. That is a choice we all have, and it must be honored.

Some of the better-known types of perception are listed below. You probably have at least a few of them, to some degree. These are also the "gifts" that I discussed in Chapter 2:

- CLAIRCOGNIZANCE: The ability to acquire information intrinsically (to just know)

- TELEPATHY: The ability to send or receive thoughts to or from someone else

- PRECOGNITION: Also referred to as second sight, prophecy, or precognition; the ability to perceive future events

- AURAS: The ability to detect energy fields around other living beings, often as white light or colored bands of energy

- CLAIRSENTIENCE: The ability to feel the emotions that others are experiencing (also referred to as empathy)

- MENTAL IMAGING: The ability to perceive another person's thoughts or mental pictures

Other common perceptual abilities, which later chapters will cover in more detail, include

- DOWSING: The ability to locate water, metals, or information by using a variety of devices

- ENERGY MEDICINE: The ability to perceive a wide variety of energies through one's hands, such as osteopathic manipulation, and utilize those perceptions in the service of healing

- CLAIRAUDIENCE: The ability to acquire information through sound waves

There are many more named abilities, many of which are beyond the scope of this book. It is my intention to focus on the most common and relatable perceptions that are most likely to enhance one's life and the ability to communicate better with others.

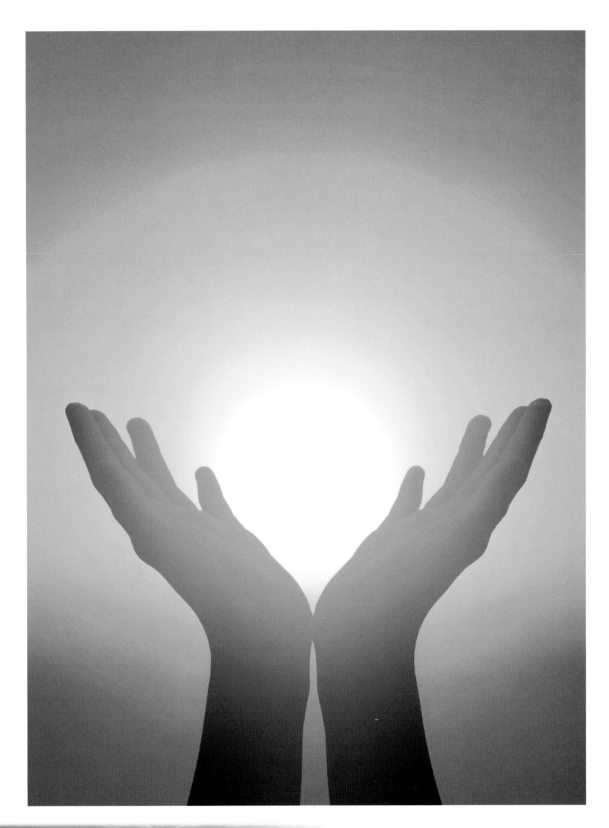

CHAPTER 5:
Important Energetic Perceptions

I have learned that making patients comfortable is critical to giving them the space to open up, express themselves, and reflect on their experiences without fear of judgment or criticism. This is much harder to do than you might think, because it requires that a practitioner be open themselves, and be honest with themselves about their likes, dislikes, and ideals. A patient can feel, immediately, how you are viewing them and will not be forthcoming if they notice any hint of discomfort on your part as their practitioner.

It may take years of self-examination, meditation, or therapy for a physician to acquire this sense of openness, which is essential to gaining a patient's trust and willingness to really work with you.

As an example, in the early years of my practice, I trained in Reichian therapy, a process developed by the eminent psychiatrist Wilhelm Reich in the 1930s and 1940s. Essentially, this training involved asking my patients to breathe in specific patterns while I observed and loosened up the tight areas of their musculature. Reich discovered that blocked emotions were held in certain muscles, and as those muscles released their tension, the corresponding emotions would be released as well.

It was a powerful process, and it helped many of my patients access emotional events that they had long repressed, enabling them to free up the energies that were tied to holding back those emotions. It turns out that repressing emotion takes a lot of energy. Once my patients released those energies, they regained their natural equilibrium and became psychologically and physically healthier.

Performing Reichian therapy required me to become more comfortable with patients who needed to release emotions so that I could create a safe space for them to do so. This simultaneously required me to become more comfortable with my own emotions; otherwise, my discomfort with emotional expression would have greatly inhibited my patients' experience.

ENERGY CORDS

I often noticed that during the emotionally charged experience of undergoing Reichian therapy, many of my patients would literally re-experience a past traumatic event. Some of them seemed to be stuck in those events by energetic connections to people who had hurt them in some way. I began to think of these as "energy cords"— threads of energy that tethered my patients to those individuals. (As I will explain a bit later in the chapter, not all energy cords are negative, but those are the ones I am speaking of here.) Because this manifestation was so strong, it seemed to me that, in order to begin true healing, they needed to remove the cord of energy that connected them to the hurtful person in question.

I asked my patients to "feel" those cords and then grab hold of them and pull them out. Some patients had great difficulty with this visualization, and it was clear that they were making halfhearted efforts to remove the cord. When I asked them to really pull out those cords by putting more effort into it, they often experienced a dramatic emotional release that led to therapeutic breakthroughs. Sometimes it seemed as if the cord re-formed immediately after being pulled out. So I added more visualizations, which included seeing the energy cord as an electrical cord that might be found on an appliance and smashing or cutting off the plug end so that the cord could not reconnect.

Initially, I viewed this very effective process simply as a guided visualization. However, over time I began to realize that it was more than that. Although I was unable to see these cords myself (I later discovered that there are people who can), my ability to feel their presence made it clear that there really were cords of energy connecting my patients to those who had hurt them. And after removing those cords, healing could finally take place.

Since I cannot see these cords, my awareness of them was drawn by my patients' physical reactions to going through their emotional releases. They might involuntarily grab their stomach or throat (without realizing it) or tighten up their diaphragm or chest, literally pointing out to me where these cords were located.

Many, if not most, of the cords came into the solar plexus or heart area of the body, but some came into the throat, pelvis, or face. Some cords were even sneakier, coming in through the patient's back rather than the front. Sometimes we had to do extensive work to find and remove all of the cords for progress to be made. In retrospect, I realize that these areas of cord connection appear to be related to what are referred to as the chakras.

Many healing traditions recognize seven energy centers, or chakras. Those who have the gift of being able to see them often describe them as having different colors. Any blockage of energy flow through any of the chakras leads to stasis and hence to disease or a decline in health. Perhaps you can think of it as simply another way to describe how energy in the body can be blocked or sidetracked. (Many of the healing methods discussed later in this book are designed to address this disruption of energy, including acupuncture, Reiki, and osteopathic manipulation.)

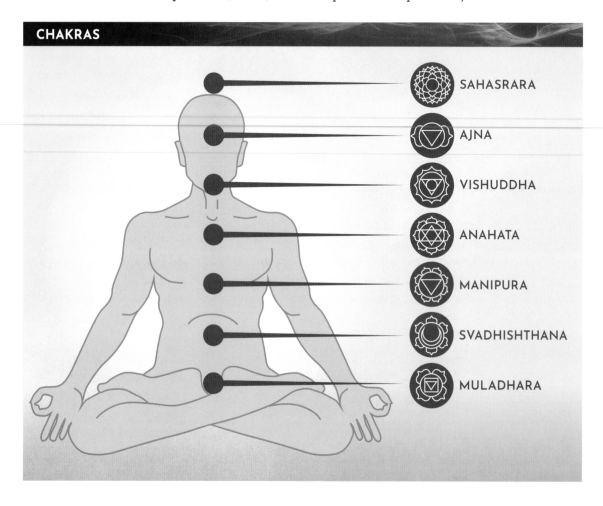

CHAKRAS

SAHASRARA

AJNA

VISHUDDHA

ANAHATA

MANIPURA

SVADHISHTHANA

MULADHARA

Some energy blockages are *internal*, meaning that some kind of traumatic stressor created the blockage. Others are *external*, meaning the blockage was caused by a connection to another person or event that holds the patient captive, even years after the experience.

- An INTERNAL BLOCKAGE might have been created by a surgical procedure. If the procedure went well, there may be no residual effects on the patient. But if the surgery was difficult, or if it led to complications such as an infection that required a prolonged hospital stay, or if it led to scarring or a fear of recurrence, an energy blockage may remain that can last for years, even though the tissues may have healed with scarring (see Chapter 9 for more on this from Dr. Dave Ou).

- An EXTERNAL BLOCKAGE may be related to a difficult interaction or communication with another person that left the patient feeling betrayed, hurt, disappointed, or angry. If those emotions are not released or worked through, an energy blockage may persist for years.

The person who caused this blockage may no longer recall the event or even be alive, but that does not matter. The patient for whom this intense experience was very real is maintaining the energy cord, and the connection persists and continues to lock up their energies and emotions.

Being aware of these energy cords so that we can help eliminate any impediments to healing that they create is a big part of energetic diagnosis. The healing that ensues when patients are liberated from these cords can be profound.

Denise Linn has an excellent description of this concept in her book *Energy Strands: The Ultimate Guide to Clearing the Cords That Are Constricting Your Life.* First, she lays out the kinds of cords, or strands, that can come into play:

- FAMILY STRANDS: parents (think umbilical cord), grandparents, siblings, aunts, and uncles

- ANCESTOR STRANDS: past generations of family members, including their teachings and attitudes

- FRIEND AND ACQUAINTANCE STRANDS

- ENEMY STRANDS: those who have meant to cause harm

- LOVER AND SEXUAL PARTNER STRANDS

- PET STRANDS

- STRANGER STRANDS

- STRANDS FROM CHILDHOOD AND THE PAST

- HEALER/THERAPIST/TEACHER/DOCTOR STRANDS

A lot of beings influence us over our lifetime. Please keep in mind that many energy cords are positive and do not need to be removed or altered in any way. Loving strands from family, friends, lovers, and pets are to be nourished. But it can be helpful to remove those cords that have left us compromised or stuck, especially those that have had a profound effect on us and are limiting our growth and ability to heal.

Of particular relevance to the subject of this book are the energy strands that can form between patient and healer/doctor. Linn writes:

> *[The creation of an energy cord] often occurs because the client forms a strong cord attachment to the healer. The loving energy of the healer flows into the client, and the pain of the client can then flow back into the healer. This same kind of attachment can occur between a client and a therapist, teacher, spiritual mentor, or doctor. If you are in a helping profession, and you feel your energy dip after working with your clients, you may want to learn how to immediately release strand attachments, so you don't take on any imbalances.*

This attaching of strands occurs far more often than most healthcare providers realize. Being aware of these strands is central to both understanding what is happening and remaining healthy by not allowing these cords to drain you.

Linn goes on to clarify the kinds of symptoms that would indicate you may have some attachments that need to be attended to, and then she provides a wide variety of techniques and approaches to help you remove those cords that are not nourishing. She then provides a variety of visualizations that you can use to better protect yourself from unwittingly attracting these cords, or when you know you are in the presence of an energy vampire or someone who may wish you harm (discussed further in Chapter 6).

The bottom line: although I began with the naïve perception that energy cords were metaphorical, it is clear to me now that they are very real.

ENERGY CORDS AS SEEKERS

We often recognize certain individuals as being unusually good at attracting good fortunes: their vacations are always blessed with great weather, they win at bingo, they seem to have the perfect spouse, or they find the perfect home. I have often referred to them as "dreamers," and the gift of dreaming is one in which those individuals appear to attract what they seek with surprising regularity. Even if dreaming is not your primary gift, your life may be affected by someone whose need is so intense that it draws you into it.

A recent example: after returning from teaching at a medical conference, I was waiting in a long line to get into an airport restaurant prior to the departure of my flight. The hostess came up to me and a gentleman standing a few yards off and apologetically asked if we would mind being seated together, as only one table was open. We looked at each other, shrugged, and took our seats.

When I travel, I usually make little effort to interact with fellow travelers, hiding in a book to minimize contact. Moreover, I do not tell those I come in contact with that I am a physician, as I really do not want to hear a litany of their medical symptoms and diagnoses or vivid descriptions of recent surgeries. Travel, for me, is a time when I can get away from the world for a little while and reflect.

Somehow, this day was different. I introduced myself, not mentioning what I did for a living, and we struck up a conversation. The man was on his way to another country for work but admitted that he had not been well for quite some time. He added that he had recently been diagnosed with mycoplasma pneumonia, a lung infection that occasionally becomes chronic, and had been wrestling with a wide variety of other symptoms.

"You wouldn't know much about it; it is a rare infection," he said. Smiling, I admitted that I might actually know quite a bit about it. And when he expressed doubt, I confessed I was a physician who had treated that particular condition for quite some time.

At that point, his demeanor changed. He became quite intense and insisted on giving me a detailed history of his condition. Again, normally I would not have solicited this information or encouraged him to share it, but something about this experience was different, and I just went with it.

Partway through his story, I realized that this man was dealing with mold toxicity, a diagnosis that no one had suggested to him; I interrupted him by guessing a wide variety of symptoms that he probably had as well. He seemed astonished, commenting, "You cannot possibly know that!"

When I explained my expertise in this area and told him that I had written several books on the subject, he almost teared up. "I prayed last night, intensely, for help," he shared. "I am so tired, and my family and company and employees need me to be healthy, but no one knows what I have or can help me. You are an answer to my prayers!" He became a bit emotional, grabbed my hand, and held it. I proceeded to go over with him how to find doctors in his area who could help him and what tests to ask for while conveying that I, indeed, understood what he had and reassured him that it could be successfully treated.

The connection between us was palpable. Our lives had come together in a way that we could not have foreseen. This chance meeting in an airport restaurant, pushed by a busy hostess to sit together—how likely was that? It turned out that neither of us believed in coincidence. What struck me most was that his intense need for help had somehow elicited a response from the universe to bring us together, for a brief moment, for healing. He had, consciously or unconsciously, sent out an energy cord into the world to which I unconsciously responded. It was a pure cord, not complicated by other agendas, but simply a cord seeking help.

He promised to follow up with me via email and let me know how he fared. I have since learned that he did make an appointment with the physician I suggested he see, and he was already making excellent progress. All I know is that this whole interaction felt right, and I found myself smiling throughout the encounter at the amazing "coincidence" that had brought us together in this unique setting.

RECOGNITION

The idea of "fate" or "divine intervention" or however we might describe energy putting us in "the right place at the right time" leads us nicely into the concept of recognition. What I mean by "recognition" is having a strong sense of connection to a person, animal, place, or event that transcends our usual way of interacting with the world.

You have probably had the experience of meeting someone for the first time and feeling, at a deep level, that you already knew them or had a connection to them. Some of the most important relationships of my life started with this kind of "aha" moment.

When I met Cheryl, the love of my life, our connection was immediate. Whether we call this love at first sight or an instantaneous awareness that "Boy, do I want to get to know this person better!" or label it in some other way, the connection is there.

Two of my longtime friendships began in a similar way. My friend and colleague Dr. Carolyn Torkelson called me over at a medical meeting in 1982 to introduce me to a young doctor she had just met, saying, "You need to meet Dr. D; he could be your brother." Dr. D (who wrote Chapter 11 of this book) and I had an immediate rapport, and we have been close friends ever since—the events of our lives have overlapped in amazing ways. At another medical meeting, I crossed the room to talk to an old friend who was conversing with another young physician, Ben Brown. Ben and I began talking, and we did not stop connecting for the entire three or four days of the conference. We too have been good friends ever since.

On a vacation in Mexico, the daughter of a friend introduced Cheryl and me to a small puppy. Feeling a similar sort of instant connection, we were drawn to find a way to bring the pup home with us. We succeeded, and Kai became an important part of our lives for fourteen years, although he surprised us by growing up to be a seventy-five-pound lap dog.

I meet new folks all the time. Many of them I like immediately, but the kind of meeting I am talking about here feels a bit different. I find this kind of connection, which I refer to as recognition, fascinating. What is it about that person that draws us to them? Do they remind us of someone else in our life who is similar? Does our subconscious recognize a similar energetic pattern or quality in the other person that grabs our attention? Some people describe this as a past life connection, and while that also may be true, I think it diminishes the immediacy of the response.

The opposite response also occurs. We can meet someone for the first time and want nothing to do with them. What is that about?

As we delve into the subject of perceiving energies, these immediate reactions should be part of the discussion. We are, physiologically, energetic beings. We constantly radiate the energetic essence of who we are to the world, whether or not we are conscious of that. We can "cloak" or "shield" that energy from others if we try, but doing so takes quite a bit of effort and can be exhausting over the long haul. And at some point, our shields will come down. I'll talk more about shielding later, but my point here is that all life forms generate an energy field, and we all are perfectly capable of picking up on and responding to those fields.

There are energy fields we are drawn to and others we are repelled by. Recognition simply refers to this process. The more we can honor our perceptions, the easier it is to make connections and widen our circle of friends. We can also protect ourselves from those who might mean us harm or might want to take some of our energy by quickly recognizing those individuals and avoiding them (that is, not coming into close enough proximity that they can affect us).

Rather than simply thinking, "Oh, that's interesting," about either a positive or a negative response to a person we've just met, we would benefit from allowing ourselves to be aware of this phenomenon of recognition and utilize it to fine-tune our relationships. Most of us already do so. The more conscious we can be of it, the better it will serve us.

CARING VERSUS COMPASSION

One of the more common difficulties that physicians, healthcare providers, and other caregivers have is understanding the difference between caring and compassion.

The word *caring* implies an act of reaching out to another being with the intent to be helpful. Along with this reaching out comes an energetic extension of your being, meaning that you are literally extending your "self" or your energy far from your body. You can visualize this as your energy field moving away from you into space to interact with another energy field. Of course, caring is laudable, but at the same time it makes your energy field vulnerable to other influences that may be in the vicinity.

To an energy vampire, which is a person who seeks to take advantage of the generosity of others without giving anything in return, this extension of your energy field is like the ringing of a dinner bell: "Come and get it!" Given the ability of energy vampires to instinctively tap into that open invitation, you are unwittingly announcing that your energy is available for the taking. Are you sure you want to do that?

Tai chi gives us the opportunity to visualize this concept in a more physical way. As tai chi students, we are taught to appreciate our movements from a place of balance. More specifically, we need to be aware of how our knees are bent as one "form" morphs into the next in the stylized dance that is tai chi. If you bend your knees too far in any movement, you are off-balance. From a martial arts perspective, being off-balance means you can be thrown or tossed easily by a practitioner who can perceive your imbalance. From a health perspective, it means you have moved your energy off of the base from which the flow of energies arises, and energy is no longer moving through your body in a healthy way.

This is not to say that caring is bad, or bad for you. Rather, to counter this open (and often unconscious) flow of energy, I suggest that *compassion* is a healthier place to come from. Compassion allows us to appreciate the difficulties or suffering that another being is experiencing and to interact with them with that understanding, but it does not require us to extend our energy field away from our bodies so that it can become compromised. It allows us to remain in balance while appreciating what another person is going through and to act accordingly—to be of help by tuning in to what that person needs and providing that assistance to the best of our ability without losing ourselves in the process.

Note how different this approach is from the usual response to finding a friend in distress and immediately saying, "You poor dear! What can I do?" This sort of reaction opens you up to being drained and depleted in a way that may not be of real help to your friend. Learning to care without extending yourself into territories in which you are vulnerable is central to being able to provide healing. Reflect on the often-used phrase "Give 'til it hurts!" Does that idea really make sense to you? Not only does it sound painful, but it doesn't even sound reasonable.

One way of describing this, and one that many traditions embrace, is that you are not intrinsically doing the healing; rather, you are allowing healing energies to come through you and flow into another person. Otherwise, you would be constantly drained and exhausted. When patients are improving, it is tempting to take credit for that improvement—our egos love it. For many years, I have used this phrase with my improving patients: "God heals. I just work here." It is a helpful way of clarifying these dynamics for the patient (and myself).

CHAPTER 6:
The Reality of Evil: There Are Those Who Wish You Harm

**SEE NO EVIL, HEAR NO EVIL, SAY NO EVIL:
A Really Bad Strategy for Protecting Yourself in the Real World**

There are, indeed, people in this world who mean you harm. We are not inclined to discuss them because we are taught that doing so makes us look petty or mean. Many spiritual teachings encourage us to turn the other cheek or to realize that those who treat us badly are simply unhappy individuals who are hurting; we should pray for them and try to understand them. We are encouraged to "give them another chance" because "they didn't really mean it."

I am going to suggest something radically different: most of the time, this empathetic approach will backfire, and you will feel even worse as you attempt to understand or help the person who seems to be affecting you adversely. This is because those who wish you harm have their own agenda. There are many names for people who can impact you in this way, but the most dramatic and accurate label in current use is "energy vampires."

To a kind, compassionate, and empathetic person, it is almost unthinkable that another person might mean them harm:

- "Surely they did not mean that mean thing they did or said."

- "I think they told me they were having a bad day."

- "I know they get this way sometimes when they are frustrated, but if I can just be patient, and love them more, and forgive them this one time, tomorrow will be better."

But it won't. Because energy vampires see life differently. Not only is it close to impossible to repair them, but they don't want to be repaired. They deeply believe that *you* are the problem. Using the time-honored methods of blame, projection, and self-absorption, they sincerely believe that they have never done anyone any wrong and their behavior is above reproach. You, however, in questioning their motives or actions, have crossed the line, and that requires an all-out attack on every aspect of your being. Everything you say is interpreted as a slight upon their character and must be rigorously discredited. *Rigorously* means "all's fair in love and war," and this is war. Energy vampires can—and will—twist the truth, exaggerate, and lie to others to present themselves as blameless and you as worthless. This is a fight you cannot win, so please do not try.

You may well have been taught that kindness will win over the hearts of those who are hurting and that, over time, they will see the light and behave better. They, on the other hand, have likely spent their lives becoming adept at identifying those tender-hearted folks whom they can use and will simply perceive you to be a foolish sucker. When you show them kindness despite their behaviors, they immediately realize that they can take advantage of you anytime they want.

I am certain that you can relate to what I have written. You have been surprised, perhaps even shocked, that someone you considered a friend turned on you in the most malevolent way. *Why? How did this happen? Am I that bad a judge of character?* And, if you are thoughtful and considerate like most of us are, you wracked your brain in an attempt to understand. You might have asked yourself: *What part did I play? What could I have done differently?* Unfortunately, you will find no answers to these questions and will simply torment yourself by trying. Anyone who acts like this has severe problems that cannot be addressed by kindness alone. To repeat, those who would treat you this way are broken. They are indeed hurting and unhappy, but they do not want to be fixed: rather, they want to take you down with them. Retribution and revenge are their mantras, even though, from your perspective, they have nothing to be vengeful about.

Your perspective, though rational, is irrelevant. Like a wounded animal, an energy vampire will lash out at the nearest target in ferocious ways. If you allow yourself to be that target, you will discover that they are relentless in their self-righteous pursuit of what they perceive as justice and and will not let go. They will make your life as miserable as their clever plans can deliver.

Here is the problem: Nice, kind, empathetic people have a great deal of difficulty believing that a person who professes love and caring is actually taking advantage of them. The delay of recognition of this harmful behavior can lead to a great deal of prolonged suffering.

Musicians recognized these energies long before psychiatrists got around to naming or labeling them. Clint Black told us, "We tell ourselves…that what we found…is what we meant to find," and, "You can't believe the things a heart can tell a mind." A beautiful way to express our unwillingness to accept that the being we want to be in love with us has another agenda, and we are going to get hurt. Kenny Rogers cautioned, "You got to know when to hold 'em, know when to fold 'em, know when to walk away, know when to run."

This is where honoring our perception of energies and emotions comes into play. Our minds are readily led astray by charismatic individuals who are adept at identifying our vulnerabilities, our need for love and appreciation, and who initially seem to know exactly what to do and say to hook us into their orbit. But, as time passes and we look at the actions of these individuals rather than their words—if we are open to it—we will see the disparities. Our feeling hearts and guts often provide this information early on in our interactions, but we are culturally taught to focus on what our minds think, not to honor the information coming from our bodies. Paying attention to what our hearts and guts are telling us allows us to see through the smoke screen, recognize what is really going on, and prevent ourselves from getting hurt and drained.

It is your energetic perception that will protect you—*if you let it.*

As a physician, I see patients stuck in relationships that drain them and hurt them emotionally and physically due to their reluctance to recognize what is happening to them. They just can't believe it, so they don't. These nice, kind, empathetic beings simply cannot wrap their minds around the fact that this energy vampire even exists, let alone could want to harm them. Or could they? I encourage all of my readers with whom this information resonates to read Dr. Christiane Northrup's excellent book *Dodging Energy Vampires* for an in-depth discussion of this subject.

If what I am describing resonates with you, you will realize that there is only one strategy for dealing with those who mean you harm: to get away from them. You cannot discuss the problem (this fuels their delusional rage), or talk about it or analyze it with them, or apologize for something you are not even sure you did. In fact, anything that reminds an energy vampire of what they think you did to them will only make them more determined to get back at you in any way they can, with the sole purpose of hurting you and making you suffer as they feel they have suffered.

All you can do to minimize the harm is to walk away and have absolutely nothing to do with that person. No contact whatsoever. Doing so helps in two ways:

- It allows you to begin the grieving process (cutting ties with someone you once loved does trigger a kind of grief) and regain the energy you lost to them.

- It takes away an easy target for the energy vampire to put their frustrations upon.

This is truly the only way you can help them. Hopefully, as they lose more and more emotional targets, they'll realize that their coping strategy is causing them harm and seek professional help (which, as Dr. Judy Tsafrir will tell us later in this chapter, is unlikely). The ideal outcome—at least for you—is that they will get bored with being angry at you and move on to someone else.

The hardest of these individuals to deal with are, understandably, those in your own family. We have been taught that "blood is thicker than water" and that no matter what, we must remain loyal to our families. My patients are commonly confused and uncertain about how to handle certain family members, be it a parent, sibling, aunt, uncle, or in-laws, when they act out at get-togethers.

After many years of enduring what is actually a form of verbal and emotional abuse, many of my patients realize that family encounters significantly set back their efforts to heal from other maladies. They leave these visits upset and hurt and, after a while, may begin to identify that one particular family member is triggering these reactions. What are they to do? Rarely can this conflict be discussed with other family members, who are often oblivious to or in denial of these behaviors and will castigate the "complainer" for even hinting that the family unit is imperfect.

As the realization sets in that every family visit is painful and troubling, even thinking about another visit triggers anxiety and stress. Are you going to be dutiful and just suck it up and somehow get through it, knowing you will spend weeks afterward recovering from the experience? Or do you have the courage to take care of yourself (which your family may call "selfish" but is really a demonstration of a good sense of self) and limit your visits, or even stop going altogether?

Here is the main thesis of this chapter: It is up to you to protect yourself. You cannot count on anyone else to do it for you. Your beloved spouse or friends may be supportive, but you have to understand the reality of what you are facing and make the healthy choice.

Especially when dealing with a dysfunctional family system, this choice can be a difficult one. Are you willing to face your family's displeasure or your own suffering? The next time you find yourself asking this question, please remember: no good will come from making others happy at the expense of your own health.

DEFINING ENERGY VAMPIRES

Understanding the pathology that underlies these behaviors will assist you in identifying those who are safe to be around and those who are not. Only by using your perceptual gifts can you be alerted early on to the presence of a difficult individual and protect yourself from that person.

In the medical field, we are increasingly using the term "energy vampires" to describe patients who interact with us in such a way that they literally take our energy from us. These are folks with whom we can spend anywhere from thirty seconds to ten minutes and feel completely drained. That drained feeling may last anywhere from hours to days.

I'm sure you have experienced this sort of interaction. You think you are having a brief, benign conversation with an acquaintance or friend, but afterward, you are surprised to find that you feel exhausted. What happened? These are people who are essentially empty inside, and they use your energy (and the energy of anyone else they come in contact with) to attempt to fill themselves. But that vessel is more like a sieve; it cannot hold your energy. Once they have sucked you dry, they will move on to someone else, forever unsatisfied, because it is an emptiness that cannot be filled.

The tip-off to recognize these individuals is easy: you feel drained. Once you have identified them, please do not attempt to fix them— you can't! You are not doing them a favor by thinking your energy will help them in any way. They will not benefit from your energy because they cannot hold on to it; it dissipates immediately. You will simply become exhausted. The strategy for dealing with these people is simple: do not go near them. No good will come of that for you or, if you are a physician treating this person, for your office staff.

Let me now speak directly to the healthcare providers among my readers. To protect yourself and your staff, please dismiss these patients as soon as possible. You cannot help them, but you can help those you care about by eliminating all contact with energy vampires. It may sound overly harsh, but I don't think that's the case. I am being realistic. If I cannot help someone, and they are toxic to me and my staff, there is no value in continuing a relationship that has no place to go. It is imperative to recognize that these folks do not want be healed despite their statements to the contrary, but they can hurt you with every contact. If you think that by continuing to try to help them, you are taking the spiritual high road, I urge you to think again. One of the spiritual gifts we are given is that of discernment, and we are always encouraged to use that perception in the service of healing. If we do not, we are turning our backs on spiritual truths and kidding ourselves about the kind of good we are doing.

The specific psychiatric diagnoses given to these patients may be in the categories of those with personality disorders, narcissists, and sociopaths. I have asked Judy Tsafrir, MD, an integrative psychiatrist who has a great deal of professional experience with this issue, to share her wisdom so we can learn how to better protect ourselves against energy vampires.

SOME REFLECTIONS ON CLINICAL VAMPIRES IN CLINICAL PRACTICE AND LIFE

by JUDY TSAFRIR, MD

The following reflections about energy vampires are based both upon my personal life experience and on my clinical experience as a psychiatrist and psychoanalyst in practice for over thirty years.

What are energy vampires? At the heart of it, they are people who do not respect the Golden Rule. They do unto others as they would never want to have done unto themselves, taking advantage of and exploiting others and typically feeling no conflict about doing so. They feel entitled to take without giving in kind, as the concept of relational mutuality or reciprocity is a foreign one. It's a one-way street, with them always on the receiving side. It's never win-win; it's win-lose. These people are often calculating, masterfully plotting to turn every situation to their advantage. Energy vampires exhibit a spectrum of behaviors, from extraordinary drama, self-centeredness, irrationality, and volatility to frank aggression and sociopathy.

Energy vampires have what psychiatry defines as a personality disorder, which is a condition that affects the way a person thinks, behaves, or relates to other people. In the *Psychiatric Diagnostic Manual,* they fall into "Cluster B," which encompasses a wide variety of conditions that usually cause more distress to others than to the individuals diagnosed with those conditions. It is unusual for an energy vampire to seek help from a psychiatrist. Patients generally seek psychological help because they are suffering and have a sense that something about the way they are approaching life is causing them pain. Energy vampires don't look at things that way. They do not believe they have a problem, but rather are masters of externalization and foisting blame on others. It's always everyone else's fault. If they do make an appointment with a mental health professional, it is usually done under duress, typically because someone has given them an ultimatum (for example, that the relationship is over if they continue to refuse treatment). As you can imagine, this is not a winning setup for successful psychotherapy.

If the energy vampire does engage, it's not uncommon for this sort of patient to attempt to victimize the practitioner. All practitioners need to be wary of the seduction of these types of patients who know just how to flatter the practitioner, which can cloud sound clinical judgment. Energy vampires can be demanding and without respect for boundaries or limits. Refusing to honor cancellation policies or pay their bills, expecting special treatment, and demanding unlimited access are regular features. It is prudent for the practitioner to be very cautious about accepting patients with this sort of character into their practice. It is not uncommon for them to eventually threaten to complain to the Board of Registration in Medicine about feeling harmed in order to get their way. This behavior is often motivated by a wish to avoid paying the bill. The board typically investigates all complaints, no matter how spurious, which creates anxiety, aggravation, and sometimes legal expense for the practitioner. At risk management seminars for psychiatrists, we have been advised not to pursue payment that is legitimately owed in order to avoid the threat of malpractice, even if the claim is baseless.

In romantic relationships, energy vampires can be very charming, often love-bombing their victims during courtship. They have an uncanny and malignant intuition about the vulnerabilities of their victims and know precisely what they need to say or do to exert influence and get their way. Many of these individuals are charismatic, professionally successful, good-looking, and sexually skilled and present themselves as larger than life. The victim is recruited to provide narcissistic supplies to buttress the fragile self-esteem of the energy vampire. If they fail to provide these supplies, they are often subject to intense negativity, criticism, and rage.

It is much more common for the victims of energy vampires to seek help than the energy vampires themselves. The patient is often the adult child of a narcissistic parent, and having their basic needs for love and respect ignored, their feelings invalidated, and their boundaries violated is absolutely familiar and feels like home. They often grew up in households where, when they expressed a need or feeling, they were accused of selfishness and hypersensitivity and were rewarded for surrendering to caretaking of the self-absorbed parent. They are used to trying to win love through service and sacrifice. The strategies of service and sacrifice, when given to an energy vampire, do not work, and when the patient persists in providing these energies, they simply get depleted and receive no recognition for these efforts. It is unlikely that they will be able to heal without minimizing their contact with the energy vampire or ending the relationship altogether. A patient can have a pristine diet, take an array of high-quality supplements, exercise religiously, sleep well, attend acupuncture and massage sessions regularly, and have meaningful work, a developed spiritual practice, and supportive family, friends, and community, but if they are in a toxic relationship, they will not feel well. Here is an example from my practice:

CASE STUDY

Loni was a forty-year-old woman who came to see me because of severe anxiety, depression, and insomnia. She had been married for seven years to an unscrupulous wealthy real estate developer ten years younger than herself. She slavishly served him, anticipating and attending to his every need, trying desperately to get him to respond to her in a loving, caring way, just as she had tried in vain to get her narcissistic mother to acknowledge and be kind to her. In return for her efforts with her husband, she had developed severe chronic pain and fatigue, which was diagnosed as fibromyalgia.

Though she enjoyed their lavish lifestyle, she recounted with embarrassment stories about her husband bullying hostesses in restaurants, claiming that they had lost his reservation when he never had one in the first place, until they finally capitulated and gave him a table. Once, when he scratched his car in a parking garage, he claimed that the damage was due to the carelessness of the valet and demanded that the restaurant where he subsequently dined pay for the repair. He threatened to sue his dentist in order to avoid responsibility for a bill for extensive dental work. Aggressive browbeating and intimidation of others resulted in him almost always getting his way.

My patient became more and more debilitated over the course of her marriage to him. When he eventually took up with a much younger woman and announced on Valentine's Day that he wanted a divorce, she was heartbroken. She reported with shock that he had suggested dividing up their possessions there and then. I was hardly surprised; it sounded consistent with everything that had preceded it. They divorced, and she moved to the other side of the country to start a new life. When I received a card from her a year later, she related that her depression, anxiety, pain, and fatigue had quickly evaporated once she was free of this man. She wrote that she was training for a marathon and felt like a new person.

As dramatic as it sounds, this is not an uncommon story, insofar as a toxic relationship can totally undermine a person's health and well-being. It is not uncommon for patients who are partnered with energy vampires to receive prescriptions for antidepressant and anti-anxiety medications because those medications can numb the distress of being in a relationship in which one is regularly subjected to manipulation, criticism, deception, and disappointment. The medications can increase the tolerance for abuse. When a patient stops these medications, they often are unable to continue putting up with the mistreatment.

If a victim of an energy vampire has the futile hope that the relationship can be salvaged and improved and persuades the partner to go to couple's therapy, it is important that the therapist be aware of the relationship dynamic between energy vampires and their victims. Many in the mental health field do not understand this relationship, ascribe to the adage "It takes two to tango," and treat the couple as though the responsibility for the dysfunction is equally shared. They do not recognize that one member of the couple is much more damaged and damaging than the other. It is crucial that the therapist not add insult to injury by recommending even more accommodating behavior by the victim.

I have seen patients whose couple's therapist had recommended that the victim continually accede to the energy vampire partner's unreasonable demands and version of reality in order to keep the peace. This advice is destructive and further erodes the victim's battered self-esteem. One patient resolved to try this strategy, consciously agreeing repeatedly to what she knew to be untrue and ridiculous just to avoid conflict. This strategy worked as long as the disagreements were between her and her husband, but when his abusive and delusional behavior and accusations extended to and involved their children, she could no longer acquiesce and felt compelled to separate from him. Sometimes in situations like these, when an energy vampire has left the relationship, they vow revenge and begin a campaign to punish the partner who will no longer endure the abuse. Energy vampires in these situations often use their children, sometimes effectively, to cause alienation from the victim parent. They attempt to manipulate the children to take their side by twisting the truth and overtly lying, painting the victim as the cause of this family distress. I have witnessed terrible psychological damage done to children by the vendetta waged by the energy vampire parent against the parent who initiated the marital separation.

It is a good outcome when the experience of victimization by the energy vampire catalyzes spiritual and psychological growth in the victim once they are able to acknowledge what has gone on and are no longer willing to participate in this dynamic. In these cases, the victim becomes empowered and is no longer willing to endure being treated in a way that they would ever treat someone else. The omnipotent fantasy from childhood is relinquished (i.e., that if they just try hard enough, their devotion and sacrifice will heal the dysfunctional parent and persuade that parent to love and care for them appropriately). When they finally recognize that they will never be able to change the energy vampire into a respectful, reasonable, and loving partner, family member, friend, or boss, they are freed. Paradoxically, acknowledging the limits of their power is what's empowering and represents a profound psycho-spiritual maturation. When all is said and done, energy vampires can be spiritual teachers, offering their victims profound lessons in seeing things for what they are and catalyzing personal growth and self-love.

You can see that this type of relationship dynamic causes a great deal of stress, anxiety, and depression in the victim, which can have a profound impact on the immune, endocrine, and nervous systems. The prolonged stress of dealing with an energy vampire can sensitize the immune system, causing over-reactivity and resulting in an autoimmune response, or it can suppress the immune system, rendering an individual particularly vulnerable to infections and toxins. Chronic stress causes cellular inflammation. It is rare that I see a patient with severely compromised immunity who does not report high levels of stress in the present, the past, or both. It is most often related to childhood trauma but can also be due to stress in adulthood. When a patient is regularly victimized by an energy vampire, it is essential to treatment that they fully grasp what is happening to them so that they can seek freedom and health.

TRUST YOURSELF, PLEASE

As you reflect on these thoughts, consider how you react when you first meet someone. If your immediate reaction is negative, how do you work with that? Have you been taught to give the person another chance? Perhaps you've been told not to judge others, or perhaps you have learned that someone who is spiritually attuned should examine themselves and find a way to accept, even love, that person despite misgivings.

Why don't you trust your own intuition? Part of the message of this chapter—the bottom line, if you will—is that you have hard-wired instinctual knowledge that is designed to protect you. You are capable of learning and recognizing energies that may be harmful and hence are to be avoided. I would submit to you that your immediate reaction, sense, or "vibe" is correct 99 percent of the time. So, how many bad experiences do you need to have with this individual whom you are not drawn to (or are actually repelled by)? How many stressful situations should you put yourself through to confirm your original perceptions? At the risk of being wrong 1 percent of the time, you will correctly protect yourself far, far, more often. Is there a voice in your head that is chastising you because you are being unfair to that 1 percent? Do you realize that you are subjecting yourself to a barrage of unpleasant, stressful, and taxing experiences that drain your precious energies? Please think about it. Protect yourself, and above all, trust yourself.

Alternatively, are you immediately charmed by a person you meet? Are they wonderfully attentive, hanging on your every word? Are they too good to be true? As you are enchanted by them, do you find yourself excusing bad behaviors that pop up unexpectedly or writing off how that person treats others? While they continue to charm you, do you inexplicably find yourself depleted rather than energized after each encounter? These are clues to listen to, so I will repeat: please protect yourself, and above all, trust yourself and your observations.

Judy Tsafrir, MD, is a board-certified holistic adult and child psychiatrist and psychoanalyst in private practice in Newton, Massachusetts, with an academic appointment at Harvard Medical School. Her approach is dedicated to healing through the integration of body, mind, heart, spirit, and environment. She is also an activist, painter, evolutionary astrologer, and Tarot reader. She can be contacted through her website, www.JudyTsafrirMD.com.

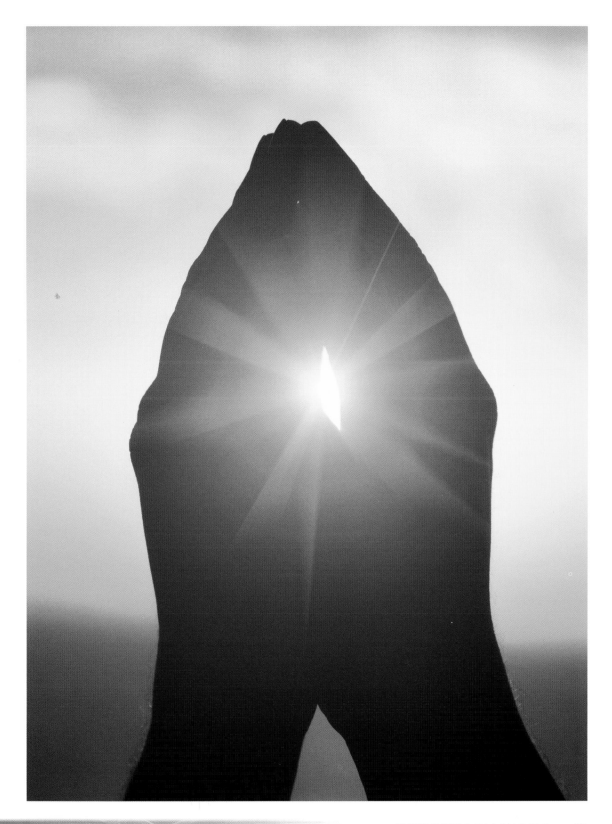

PART II
The Detection of Energy by Humans and Medical Devices and Its Medical Uses

Let's shift gears a bit and explore how perceptions of energy can be utilized more specifically in the service of diagnosis and treatment. In Chapter 7, I will briefly review the medical devices that use different types of energetic perception to provide unique treatments. After initially labeling many of these devices as having little value and possibly being harmful, the medical profession has slowly begun to embrace some of them as helpful for treating a variety of medical conditions, and a growing number of these devices are now in common use. It is my intention not to provide an encyclopedic review but to give an overview of devices and efforts to utilize energy for diagnosis and treatment.

An excellent overview of the importance of energies in diagnosis and healing can be found in the tenth anniversary edition of the landmark book *The Biology of Belief*, by Bruce Lipton, PhD (www. brucelipton.com). On page 88, he reminds us that:

> *Quantum physicists discovered that physical atoms are made up of vortices of energy that are constantly spinning and vibrating; each atom is like a wobbly spinning top that radiates energy. Because each atom has its own specific energy signature (wobble), assemblies of atoms (molecules) collectively radiate their own identifying energy patterns. So every material structure in the universe including you and me, radiates a unique energy signature.*

Later, on page 99, he goes on to say:

> *Hundreds upon hundreds of other scientific studies over the last fifty years have consistently revealed that "invisible forces" of the electromagnetic spectrum profoundly impact every facet of biological regulation. These energies include microwaves, radio frequencies, the*

visible light spectrum, extremely low frequencies, acoustic frequencies, and even a newly recognized form of force known as scalar energy. Specific frequencies and patterns of electromagnetic radiation regulate DNA, RNA, and protein syntheses; alter protein shape and function; and control gene regulation, cell division, cell differentiation, morphogenesis (the process by which cells assemble into organs and tissues), hormone secretion and nerve growth and function. Each one of these cellular activities is a fundamental behavior that contributes to the unfolding of life. Though these research studies have been published in some of the most respected mainstream biomedical journals, as of 2010 their revolutionary findings have not been incorporated into the medical school curriculum.

On page 100, he adds:

We know that living organisms must receive and interpret environmental signals in order to say alive. In fact, survival is directly related to the speed and efficiency of signal transfer. The speed of electromagnetic energy signals is 186,000 miles per second, while the speed of a diffusible chemical is considerably less than one centimeter per second. Energy signals are a hundred times more efficient and infinitely faster than physical chemical signaling.

Dr. Lipton is emphasizing the relevance and importance of energy signaling in our day-to-day functioning, so it is clearly important that we bring some discussion of it to the fore.

In Chapter 8, we will turn to one of the most versatile and effective treatments that I have found: Frequency Specific Microcurrent (FSM). Then we will move on to kinesiology and related diagnostic processes such as A.R.T. in Chapter 9. Chapter 10 discusses Reiki, and Chapter 11 moves on to dowsing and sound therapy. We will discuss the age-old healing process of acupuncture and the osteopathic cranial approach in Chapters 12 and 13, respectively. And in the last chapter of Part II, my physician-brother, Gene Nathan, MD, shares the insights he has gained through his many years of study of the healing properties of dreaming.

I have asked some of the best practitioners of these disciplines to write a few of these chapters because their expertise in these areas far exceeds mine. To help you better relate to these diagnostic and treatment procedures, I requested that they relay their experiences with these methods in as personal a way as possible. I believe this will help you understand how important it is for these wonderful physicians to use their individual abilities to perceive these energies and their intuition to improve their patients' healing results.

CHAPTER 7:

The Use of Medical Devices to Perceive Energy

One of the first big steps in the early evolution of humankind was the development of the ability to use fire for warmth, cooking, and protection. In 63 AD, Scribonius Largus, physician to Julius Caesar, reportedly discovered that electrical stimulation, in the form of standing on electrically charged fish on the seashore, could be used to relieve pain.

In the late 1700s and into the next century, the fascination with electrical devices grew, and a host of unusual contraptions were brought forth as potentially beneficial for a variety of medical conditions. It is not clear to what extent these inventions were helpful or harmful, but the effort to harness electricity for healing reached a peak in the 1920s. Albert Abrams produced one of the most popular of these devices that purportedly detected unbalanced electrical fields in a human body and treated them via a process called radionics. Radionics was controversial; some physicians felt that this method was indeed useful for both diagnosis and treatment, but eventually the governing bodies of medicine labeled it quackery, and it fell into disuse. For decades, a skeptical eye was cast upon all electrical inventions reported to provide health benefits.

The tide began to turn when, in 1974, neurosurgeon C. Norman Shealy developed the TENS (Transcutaneous Electrical Nerve Stimulation) unit and showed it to have clear benefits in the relief of pain. Dr. Shealy took this technology a step further and demonstrated that in patients with severe pain who could not be helped by medications or other modalities, he could implant the electrodes that carried this type of current into the spine to relieve pain and allow these patients to become more functional. The spinal stimulator is still in use, with the latest electrical devices and surgical procedures improving on the original model.

THE TENS UNIT: TRANSCUTANEOUS ELECTRICAL NERVE STIMULATION

The TENS unit is a flexible device that can be programmed to deliver electrical energy in a variety of wave forms and stimulation ranging from 2 to 200 hertz (Hz). Some patients respond to lower frequencies and others to higher frequencies, which corresponds to how the body produces different neurotransmitters. It is thought to work through several mechanisms, all of which involve the modulation or suppression of pain signals. It can inhibit pain signals originating from the spinal cord and can stimulate the body's production of natural opioids, such as endorphins, enkephalins, and dynorphins.

The practitioner simply places self-sticking electrodes over the parts of the body that warrant stimulation. Those electrodes are attached by wires to a small battery-powered unit that easily attaches to a belt. The patient turns a dial on the unit so that they barely feel the current, and it can be worn for long periods. Running the electrical current specifically through an acupuncture meridian and placing an electrode over the meridian above and below the area of pain can augment the treatment using the healing principles of acupuncture. In acupuncture, pain is thought to be caused by a blockage of energy flow through an area of the body, and by stimulating energy to move through that blocked area, pain can be relieved. (See Chapter 12 for more on acupuncture.)

As an example of using TENS in the treatment of low back pain (one of the most common issues seen in physicians' offices), the practitioner would place four electrode pads on the patient's body, two each about an inch away from the spine, above the area of pain, and two below the area of pain. In acupuncture terms, the electrode placement would correspond to the bladder meridian, a major pathway of energy flow that corresponds anatomically to the lower back region and runs down the back in the same way that the sciatic nerve does. The patient would then simply turn on the unit and allow it to operate for as long as desired.

My professional use of TENS allowed several instances of dramatic pain relief that demonstrated to me just how effective it can be. As background, I first studied acupuncture in 1975 with a Chinese acupuncturist who worked one day a week in our clinic in northern California. Initially, only needles were used. When TENS appeared, under the tutelage of Dr. Shealy, with whom I worked for many years, attaching the TENS unit to the acupuncture needles provided a very effective treatment. By 1985, having used TENS in the hospital-based pain clinic where I was the medical director, I had been approached by several patients who were unable to take anesthesia because of the severe reactions they'd had to it. Each of these patients had severe jaw pain and was scheduled to have surgery to repair their jaw but did not know how they could undergo the surgery given the limitations of not being candidates for anesthesia. Having heard that acupuncture could be used for anesthesia, they wanted me to try acupuncture needles attached to a TENS unit. Although I had been doing acupuncture for many years by then, I confess that both I and the surgeon who performed these surgeries were astonished by the effectiveness of using TENS with acupuncture to block these patients' jaw pain. The surgeries proceeded smoothly, without difficulty, using this type of anesthesia alone.

CES (CRANIAL ELECTRICAL STIMULATION)

There are limitations and contraindications for the TENS unit. It is not to be used directly over the eyes or anywhere on the head, for example. In the mid-1980s, Saul Liss, PhD, developed the CES (Cranial Electrical Stimulation) device, which delivers electrical impulses through two ear clips. Using much higher frequencies than the TENS unit (15,000 Hz), it delivers two slightly different waves, just a few hertz apart, to the body simultaneously; the difference in frequencies allows the impulses to enter the body as a "carrier wave." CES turned out to be an effective method that can be used on the head for both pain relief and the treatment of depression. Dr. Liss worked with Dr. Shealy and published a series of papers demonstrating a marked increase in serotonin, endorphins, cortisol, and GABA following this type of stimulation. The FDA has determined that these devices, which do not require the use of needles, are effective for the treatment of pain, depression, anxiety, and insomnia.

Dr. Shealy, who was already a leader in the treatment of pain, then established one of the first pain clinics to offer a more comprehensive treatment for chronic pain. This included the use of his TENS unit along with extensive physical therapy, psychotherapy, occupational therapy, and the use of biofeedback devices. When combined, these treatments revolutionized our approach to chronic pain, and to this day it is the model used throughout the United States.

BIOFEEDBACK

Biofeedback is another example of how a device can be used to measure and modify a physiological process in the service of healing. The impetus for the integration of different types of biofeedback came in 1964 from the work of Elmer Green, MD, at the Menninger Clinic in Topeka, Kansas (which has since been relocated to Houston, Texas). Dr. Green built a device that measured the tension in muscles and informed the patient wearing the device about how much tension was present in those muscles via earphones that registered this tension as a clicking or whining sound. When the whining or clicking increased, the tension in the muscles was higher, and when it reduced in intensity, the muscles were more relaxed. Being hooked up to muscle-tension biofeedback devices, patients with pain were able to learn with more precision how much tension they were holding, and it empowered them to relax those muscles, which led to a decrease in pain. Originally used for muscle-tension headaches with great success, it benefited most pain patients whose muscles tightened up in response to their pain. As physicians, we could tell our patients that they needed to relax, but in reality, they had no idea how to do it. Now we had a method to accomplish just that.

As the appreciation of biofeedback as an effective medical treatment evolved, the medical community realized that other physiological perceptions in the body could be measured, and that information could be fed back to patients so they could learn to modify their physiology. Biofeedback allowed a patient to simply tape an electrode that measured temperature to their finger, and that temperature would appear on a dial that the patient could monitor. One of the first conditions shown to respond to this kind of feedback was migraine headaches. Migraine patients are prone to cold hands and feet, which are an indicator of poor blood flow to those areas. In fact, many migraine patients have a finger temperature reading of 70 degrees or less. (Normally, it would be above 90 degrees.) When given the opportunity to monitor the temperature of their fingers and given relaxation skills that would increase blood flow (and hence warm up their fingers), these patients learned, over several sessions, that they could raise their finger temperature to 90 degrees in just a few minutes. By doing so, they could prevent or treat their headaches effectively without the use of medications.

Another area that is easily monitored is heart rate. In simple terms, an elevated heart rate reflects an overexcited sympathetic nervous system, usually from tension, stress, or anxiety. A lower heart rate reflects a more relaxed state. But, as it turns out, it is not that simple. A phenomenon called *heart rate variability* (HRV) reflects the ability of the nervous system to be flexible and adapt to the environment in the moment. This means that if we are emotionally upset, an electrocardiogram will show a decrease in the variability of our pattern. If we are relaxed and comfortable, the pattern becomes more variable, which is referred to as a coherent heart rhythm pattern. This is an excellent descriptor of an autonomic system in balance.

In 1991, Doc Childre formed the HeartMath Institute to further this concept. HRV is now used by physicians in hundreds of clinics around the world as an accessible form of biofeedback to help patients get their autonomic nervous systems back into balance. It can be measured by devices in an office setting, but it is more common to use an app for your phone or smart watch that shows you what kind of heart rate patterns you are having and then employ a variety of breathing techniques to bring it into coherence.

Neurofeedback followed. As another form of biofeedback, neurofeedback involves using a device to measure brain waves, which are electrical signals from the brain. That information is fed back to the patient visually or by sound. Patients can learn how to modify their brain waves based on this feedback, and this is of great benefit for a wide variety of neurological conditions, including ADHD, dyskinesias, tremors, and traumatic brain injury (TBI). While there are many forms of neurofeedback, one device that has been of particular benefit to my patients is the LENS.

THE LENS: LOW ENERGY NEUROFEEDBACK SYSTEM

Most of the biofeedback I have been discussing involves finding some way to obtain information about a specific biological function (for example, muscle tension, temperature, blood flow, or brain waves) and teaching a patient how to alter that information (such as by reducing muscle tension or increasing temperature). What makes the LENS unique is that the patient does not have to be aware of the information being processed and does not need to cooperate or work at learning a new skill, which can be very difficult for patients with cognitive impairment.

To utilize the LENS, a sensor is attached to each ear and another to the scalp. No needles are used. The information detected by the sensors is fed (via an electroencephalogram, or EEG, device) into a computer that analyzes the brain waves from twenty-one different locations in the brain, a program referred to as brain mapping. The resonant, always-changing feedback is relayed to the computer through the EEG, and the computer "reads" these signals and literally "maps" out the brain wave pattern. When the computer completes this analysis, looking for areas of the brain in which the brain waves are diminished, it provides feedback (which is not volitional on the part of the patient) in the form of a tiny (almost homeopathic) electrical signal that allows the brain waves to be, in a sense, redirected, creating a literal "reboot" of the nervous system.

For example, just recently, a patient of mine who had Lyme disease and had been worried about her cognitive decline (she was concerned that it was Alzheimer's dementia) was treated with her second session of the LENS. Within moments of her treatment, she was delighted to discover that her mind was much clearer and her thinking had dramatically improved along with her memory. This shift not only held but continued to improve with subsequent treatments.

The LENS is especially helpful for those individuals who are unable to think clearly because their brains have been damaged or are inflamed by toxins or infections. Most notably, this includes people on the autism spectrum (which includes Asperger's syndrome and ADHD) and those with TBI, bipolar disorder, chemotherapy- or chemically induced cognitive impairment, epilepsy, stroke, anxiety, depression, Tourette's disorder, post-traumatic stress disorder (PTSD), Parkinson's disease, dyskinesias, pseudo-seizures, and early-stage Alzheimer's disease. What all of these conditions share, when uncomplicated by other medical issues, are variants of one fundamental process—*how the brain tries to cope with actual or potential irritability and/or inflammation*. Because of the enormous variety of ways in which an individual's brain can develop, these conditions may present differently in different people.

Dr. Len Ochs, who developed the LENS, believes that the inability to think clearly is partly the effect of the underlying medical condition, but also the result of how the brain attempts to cope with actual or even anticipated brain irritability. Brain irritability, closely linked to inflammation, can be caused by injury, chemical or heavy metal toxicity, or infections. The brain seems to try to deal with the spread of this electrical irritability both by chemically dampening that activity (electrical suppression) and by creating "firewalls" across the surface and within the tissues of the brain to prevent those irritable signals from spreading.

While these processes are natural, they interfere with the kinds of communication the brain needs to function properly. Some people recover from this altered neurochemistry when the brain puts out the "all clear" signal that the danger has passed. However, others cannot refresh their neurochemistry or reboot the connections in their brains, and they may remain functionally impaired for life. The LENS, using extremely weak but precisely directed electrical signals (based on the brain-wave analysis obtained from brain mapping), appears to catch the brain's attention and interrupt its repetitive but nonproductive attempts to block its own communications so that it can resume more normal functioning.

Since learning of the LENS, I have found it be a superb and safe tool for patients whose brain fog and cognitive impairment prevent them from functioning properly. For example, a young man came to our clinic several years ago after sustaining a brain injury requiring hospitalization for a coma that lasted several weeks. This injury, which had occurred two years before we initially saw him, had left him exhausted and without the ability to think or express himself clearly. It had also led to intense depression and mood swings and a fear that he would never recover. Within two months of starting LENS treatments, he reported 60 to 70 percent improvement, after having made little to no progress over the preceding two years despite a variety of other treatments. His depression and mood swings were now gone, his energy had improved, and he was able to think much more clearly, enough that he was able to resume college classes.

Of particular relevance for my unusually sensitive patients, many of whom have Lyme disease or mold toxicity, is that many of these individuals have residual neurological problems even after their toxicity and/or infections have resolved. These neurological symptoms include dystonias (odd, uncontrollable writhing motions of the arms and legs), pseudo-seizures, tics, and spasms. The continuation of these symptoms even after the underlying illness has been properly addressed confuses both patients and practitioners. The patients appear to be stuck in an electrical pattern that their bodies seem unable to fix. The LENS has proven an effective tool for many of them.

OTHER ENERGY-BASED THERAPIES

As the medical profession began to utilize more energy-based therapies, those approaches became more refined and effective. For example, electroconvulsive therapy (ECT) began to be used in the 1930s as a desperate effort to help patients who were severely depressed to the point of feeling suicidal. With little else to offer patients, doctors found ECT to be effective often enough to justify its use. However, the early efforts used high doses of electricity, without anesthesia, and were often associated with severe memory loss or broken limbs from patients thrashing around while being shocked.

ECT's reputation was further damaged by the publication of Ken Kesey's book *One Flew Over the Cuckoo's Nest* in 1962, followed by the popular movie in 1975. While the concerns expressed in that book were valid, it is sometimes overlooked that there were few alternatives at the time, and those concerns resulted in an improvement in ECT procedure: it began to be done only under general anesthesia and with much lower doses of electricity. Essentially, the patient is sedated and brought to a quiet, equipped room. Electrodes are placed on their scalp, and electrical current is passed through the brain area. The patient is gently restrained, as the passage of current may cause involuntary contraction of the patient's muscles.

ECT thus became much safer and is still used as an option for treating those with severe or treatment-resistant depression, mania, catatonia, and aggression and agitation in some patients with dementia. More recently, neurosurgeons and neurologists have developed other, more precise tools to help these patients.

The deep brain stimulator, long used to help patients with Parkinson's disease control their tremors, is now being used for depression as well. In this procedure, a neurosurgeon runs electrodes into Brodmann Area 25 of the brain. This is an area of the cerebral cortex closely associated with sadness and depression. Electrical stimulation has been effective for improving depression in those who have not responded to any other type of treatment.

Another recent, less invasive development is the use of transcranial magnetic stimulation (TMS). In this procedure, an electromagnetic coil is applied against the scalp near the forehead; it has been shown to be an effective tool for some patients with treatment-resistant depression.

Most of what I have described thus far involves the use of electrical energy to monitor and treat a variety of medical conditions. This is not intended to be a comprehensive discussion of these devices, some of which are high-tech, but merely a sampling. I hope it begins to convey to you that medical science has embraced the concept of treatments that involve the use of energy, and by expanding our discussion, we can enhance our diagnostic and therapeutic options to a greater degree.

Sound and light are being utilized in this fashion as well. Two books by Norman Doidge, MD, *The Brain's Way of Healing* and *The Brain That Changes Itself,* call attention to groundbreaking research in the field of neuroplasticity. It has long been held in neurology that once the brain has been damaged, little can be done to repair it. Neuroplasticity refers to the growing realization that the synapses of the brain can shift and change in response to a wide variety of stimuli, and therefore the brain can create new pathways that allow the body to function at much higher levels.

In his books, Dr. Doidge reviews the research of Fred Kahn, MD, a vascular surgeon who became fascinated by the healing effects of specific frequencies or wavelengths of light. Dr. Kahn spent years developing BioFlex Laser Therapy, which first utilizes red light frequencies to prepare the tissues of the body for deeper healing, and then uses infrared frequencies (which penetrate deeper into the tissues) to decrease inflammation, swelling, and pain. Dr. Doidge also describes the PoNS (portable neuromodulation stimulator), which is a medical device developed at the Tactile Communication and Neurorehabilitation Laboratory at the University of Wisconsin-Madison. Essentially, the patient (with a wide variety of neurological diagnoses) holds a wafer-thin electrode on their tongue while performing specific exercises that are individualized to promote their healing. The electrode appears to send electrical stimuli to the brain, which stabilizes brain waves and allows them to fire in unison.

One of the neurological issues common to what are termed "neurodegenerative diseases" (which include such diagnoses as Alzheimer's disease, Parkinson's disease, multiple sclerosis, and autism) are what Dr. Doidge calls "noise." When neurological tissues become inflamed or overstimulated, they fire more randomly, and the brain is unable to make sense of this electrical noise. Getting the neurons back into a state of entrainment, in which the synapses of the brain are firing in a more coherent pattern, allows healing to take place. Combined with the electrical stimulation, the patient's rehabilitation exercises are designed to awaken the whole functional system; quiet sensory noise; and stimulate balance, motor movement, and mental focus.

Dr. Doidge goes on to describe the remarkable work of French physician Alfred Tomatis, who discovered that sound can be used in healing the brain and nervous system. He developed the Electronic Ear, a device that allows the human ear to focus on particular sounds and filter others out. Dr. Tomatis discovered that certain sound frequencies allow the muscles of the inner ear, the stapedius and tensor tympani, to relax from a hypervigilant state, which enables more of the healing higher frequencies to be processed. This helps patients *listen* better, which in turns stimulates the brain to process information better. It has proven to be particularly effective for children with autism, ADHD, and sensory and auditory processing disorders, including dyslexia.

I hope that at this point, I have set the table for the upcoming chapters that go into more detail about these processes for treating patients with energy-based techniques. If you are like me and grew up watching *Star Trek* on television, I'm sure you can understand how I longed to see the real-life development of the tricorder that Dr. McCoy used for diagnostics. He could simply pass the device over a body and know exactly what was wrong with it and how to heal it. Perhaps that will happen in our lifetime, or maybe we will learn that we can do the same thing without the need for any device.

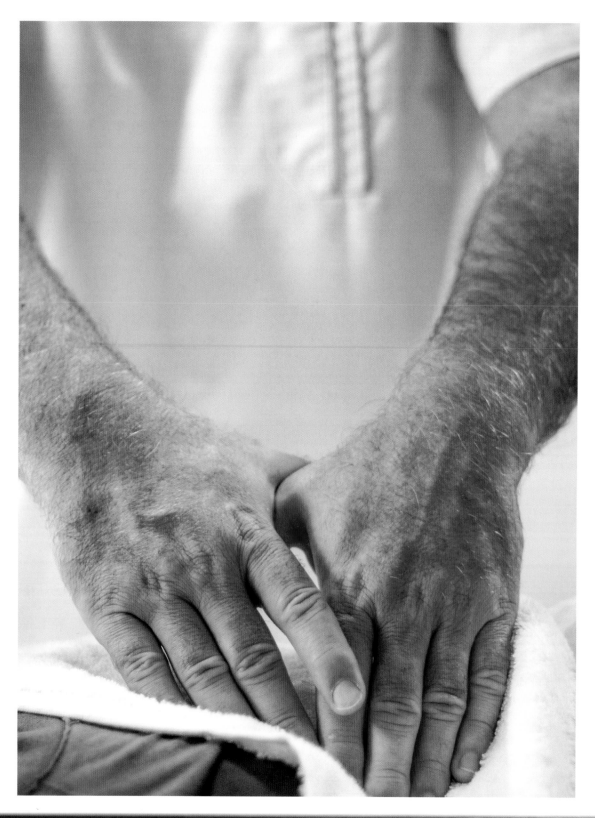

HUMAN PERCEPTIONS VERSUS ELECTRONIC DEVICES IN THE SERVICE OF HEALING

I have a personal view that I will share with you now, and it reflects the order in which I have placed the following chapters.

In my osteopathic training, I was taught that the human hand is the most sensitive diagnostic instrument available to us. While I did not fully understand the implications of that sentence when I first heard it, I have since come to believe it. Our hands are capable of tuning in to a huge spectrum of energetic information; my teachers have not only shown that this is possible but also demonstrated it to me repeatedly in my forty-year training in osteopathic manipulation. Unlike medical devices, we humans are not limited to working within the constraints of a machine. We are capable of so much more, which is the essence of this book. It is my belief that we can all tune in to the full extent of our capacities, and by doing so we enhance our ability not only to diagnose and treat, but also to appreciate the natural world and the profound energies that exist within it.

Having said this, it is also important to welcome the use of any medical device that enhances our perceptions and enables us to improve our ability to diagnose and treat.

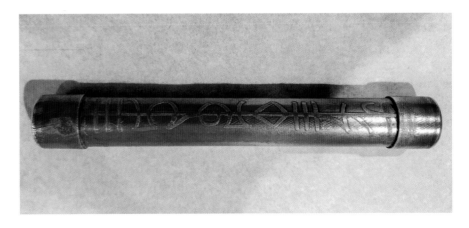

A Lemurian
Healing Rod.

CHAPTER 8:

Frequency Specific Microcurrent and Informed Intuition

"Stay Tuned to This Channel"

On my first day at work at Gordon Medical Associates in 2009, I was treated to a lecture by pioneering chiropractor Carolyn McMakin, who rediscovered and further developed the technology of Frequency Specific Microcurrent (FSM). She caught my attention when she stated that FSM could remove inflammation from the spinal cord. I was unaware that any treatment could do that. She was discussing a variant of fibromyalgia called cervical trauma fibromyalgia, which is caused by persistent inflammation in the spinal cord that follows whiplash or a head injury.

I was initially skeptical, but after using FSM to treat several of my patients (for a condition that I had not even known existed prior to this lecture), I quickly realized that not only did FSM work as advertised, but it was able to rapidly reverse long-standing physiologies in ways that nothing else I had studied ever had. And that was just the beginning. FSM turned out to be an amazingly flexible tool for the treatment of many medical conditions, and we are just scratching the surface of its potential.

Carolyn has graciously agreed to share the history of FSM and some of her findings and theories on intuitive healing here.

A BRIEF HISTORY OF FSM

by CAROLYN MCMAKIN, DC

Frequency Specific Microcurrent (FSM) is a treatment technique that uses a modern two-channel microcurrent device to deliver two different frequencies to the body at the same time. The original machine, made in 1922, was a plug-in-the-wall device. That device and its list of frequencies were rediscovered in 1946 by a British osteopath who purchased the device from its first owner, Harry van Gelder. George Douglas, DC, worked with that osteopath and brought the list of frequencies home to Portland, Oregon, in 1983. In 1995, Douglas found that list buried in a drawer and shared it with me. We wondered whether these frequencies might work on a battery-operated two-channel microcurrent machine. We started using the frequencies from the list to treat patients with difficult chronic pain with astonishing success.

Microcurrent machines deliver tiny amounts of current that the body can use directly to increase energy in cells and change cell membrane health and function. When our patients started to recover, these frequencies formed the basis of the techniques now known and taught as FSM.

Frequencies are pulses per second delivered by electrical devices or as sound. We use frequencies every day in our lives; we commonly experience them in music. When two tuning forks are placed next to each other and both are tuned to 440 hertz (Hz), they will produce the same frequency when struck. Resonance is the effect of frequencies on nearby structures. If you strike only one 440 Hz tuning fork, the fork next to it will begin to hum the same note stimulated by the vibrations or resonance of its neighbor. You can open your car door with a remote key fob that uses a frequency tuned only to your car. That's frequency specific resonance.

The frequencies that were listed on the paper Douglas rediscovered seemed straightforward enough. The first part of that list included frequencies for what we think of as pathologies that make tissues malfunction: conditions like inflammation and chronic inflammation, infections (such as viruses, bacteria, or parasites), toxins, scar tissue, and fibrosis. We now call this list of pathologies "Channel A." By stimulating these precise frequencies, Douglas and I found we could change unhealthy cell functions into healthy cell functions to relieve pain, fatigue, and illness. The second part of the list was for frequencies that are specific to tissues and organs, which make our bodies work well when they're healthy and make us feel pain, fatigued, or ill when they're not healthy. For example, we had frequencies for joints, muscles, ligaments, tendons, bones, intestines, endocrine organs, brain, and nerves. We call this list "Channel B."

That is where FSM started in 1995. The theory was that if you removed the pathology from the tissues causing pain or illness, then those tissues would return to normal healthy function and the patient would recover. Removing those conditions seems to involve the frequencies changing the cell membrane receptors, and the cell membrane receptors then act as if they change the genes inside the cells to make the cells behave more normally.

The practice of choosing the right frequencies to remove the right pathology (Channel A) from the right tissue (Channel B) turned out to be rather complicated. And explaining or teaching the practice to others was even more challenging. The frequencies turned out to be very specific and always effective as long as the patient was hydrated. New practitioners were able to achieve excellent results, but only if they knew which tissue was causing the problem and which pathology needed to be removed to make the tissue and the patient healthy again. In order to teach others to reproduce the effective treatments, I had to train them to think about how tissues really work and what really goes wrong to make tissues painful or make patients sick.

This is especially challenging when the diagnosis is not obvious. The case of the "pear-picking shoulder pain patient," whom I will call Dave, comes to mind.

By 1999, we had found that shoulder pain is pretty easy to treat with FSM. The nerves in the shoulder come from the neck and become painful when the pathology on the Channel A list called inflammation seeps out of the discs in the neck and onto the nearby nerves. Inflamed nerves from the neck create pain in the shoulder, and then the nerves tighten the shoulder muscles, changing shoulder movement and function from comfortable and smooth to painful and limited. Patients would arrive with "shoulder muscle pain," bursitis, and abnormal shoulder movement called impingement. The FSM treatment for shoulder pain usually resulted in rapid resolution of the problem. The treatment consisted of placing the microcurrent contacts on the neck and upper arm. We would remove the condition of inflammation by using 40 Hz on Channel A and treat the nerve tissue by using 396 Hz on Channel B. Reducing inflammation in the nerves consistently reduced shoulder pain and relaxed the muscles. After that, reducing inflammation in the bursa and normalizing shoulder movement was easy. It always worked—until the day it didn't.

Dave came in on a Wednesday with typical shoulder pain, abnormal shoulder movement, and bursa inflammation. His problems should have been easy to treat, but using the frequencies for inflammation in the nerves did nothing for his pain, and the tiny knots in his muscles didn't change at all. Experience told me that something else had to be the cause; intuition told me to ask more detailed questions and find out what was really going on.

Carolyn: *"How did you hurt your shoulder?"*

Dave: *"I was picking pears in my Uncle Ralph's orchard two weeks ago. That always makes my shoulder a little sore for a few days, but this time the pain didn't go away."*

C: *"Tell me about Uncle Ralph's orchard."*

D: *"We pick pears in his orchard every year at a big family potluck. After the family is finished, Ralph calls in the professionals and sends the rest of the pears to a cannery."*

C: *"You do this every year?"*

D: *"Yes. It's a great weekend. There are lots of cousins and fun, and the pears are terrific. I'm usually sore for a few days, but this year was different. I didn't get better. As a matter of fact, it's getting worse."*

C: *"What was different about this year?"*

D: *"Nothing was different. The same ladders. The same tree height. Same amount of fruit. Same number of hours picking. Same people. Same kinds of food we always eat. Same bad jokes." (He smiled as he said this and shrugged his shoulders at the happy memories.)*

That's when experience and intuition whispered into my ear: "It's never nothing." What was Dave not mentioning that could make a difference? For some reason I asked:

C: *"Does Uncle Ralph have an organic orchard? Or does he use pesticides?"*

D: *"He always uses some pesticides, but now that you mention it, this year he sprayed the pears at the very last moment you can spray them and still eat them or send them to the cannery. Last year my cousin Susan touched a spider on a pear, screamed, and almost fell off the ladder. So, this year, he sprayed a lot later than usual."*

So, one thing was different. Now I had to find out if this one change could make a difference in this particular patient. Intuition led me to ask more questions.

C: *"How does your body deal with chemicals and pesticides?"*

D: *"Not sure. How would I know?"*

C: *"Your liver has to process all sorts of chemicals that you encounter using pretty much the same enzyme detoxification pathways to do everything. So, how does your liver deal with alcohol?"*

D: *"What do you mean?"*

C: *"Can you drink your cousins under the table, or are you pretty sensitive to alcohol?"*

D: *"My cousins can drink way more than I can. I am a lightweight. One beer, glass of wine, or a mixed drink is my limit. After that I act stupid and get a hangover."*

C: *"That's one pathway. The other pathway detoxifies caffeine. How do you deal with caffeine? Can you have a cup of coffee or tea at 7 p.m. and go to sleep at 9 p.m.?"*

D: *"Nope. I can't do that either. If I have caffeine after noon, I'll be up late and have a hard time sleeping."*

There it was. The one difference in the orchard this year was the timing of the application of pesticides. And Dave didn't have a liver that detoxified chemicals very well. Now, in order to confirm this logical theory, we had to see if using different frequencies would make his shoulder better.

There are three frequencies on our Channel A list for general and organic toxins like pesticides, caffeine, and alcohol. Those frequencies are 57 Hz, 900 Hz, and 920 Hz, respectively. The tissues that are sensitive to these toxins could be the nerves, the muscles, or the fascia covering the muscle. The frequencies for reducing inflammation didn't do anything to help, so maybe the frequencies for removing toxins would help. The contacts were already in place at Dave's neck and shoulder, so it was just a matter of changing the frequencies. Using the frequencies for removing toxins from the nerves did nothing. Using the frequencies for removing toxins from the *fascia* changed everything. The fascia and the muscle relaxed; the pain disappeared; and the muscles started working together to move Dave's shoulder properly. He was pain-free in thirty minutes. The effectiveness of this treatment added weight to our explanation of how Dave had incurred his shoulder pain.

EXPERIENCE, PATTERN RECOGNITION, INTUITION, AND HEALING

It was a combination of experience and intuition that led us to choose the right frequencies to treat Dave's shoulder pain. Experience said, "The treatment for shoulders always works." Intuition said, "When the treatment doesn't work, ask questions to find out what's different and figure out what might work."

Experience teaches us pattern recognition. Pattern recognition is what tells you that when you see certain things together in one place, it means something. When you look out the living room window and see a clear blue sky above and a blanket of sparkling white covering the ground, experience and pattern recognition tell you that when you step outside, the air will be cold, and you should wear a warm jacket. When you look out the same window and see a clear blue sky and a shimmer of heat rising from the sidewalk and dusty brown grass in the yard, experience and pattern recognition tell you that a blast of hot air will greet you when you open the door, and you should wear a short-sleeve shirt and shorts.

Experience and pattern recognition depend on the observation and analysis of events and your memory of the patterns that preceded them. You see (or do) this and then that happens. Or you see this and then do that and then that happens—every time or at least most of the time. As a child, the first few times you see or do anything, you don't recognize the pattern, and you make mistakes. If you're lucky, your parents will tell you what the pattern is and how to recognize it and make the right decision. For example, this is a stove; it's hot. If you touch it, it can burn you. Don't touch it! Then you happen to touch it and it hurts, and you remember the pattern even more clearly. As you gain experience, you learn discernment. You learn that a stove can be hot, but sometimes it isn't. You learn to watch for the shimmer of heat rising from the surface or the smell of cooking food or burning wood. These are the experiences that lead to pattern recognition.

Intuition is different. Intuition seems to happen quietly inside your head. It whispers words of warning or shows you soft visions of what might be ahead for senses that aren't concrete like sight or hearing. Intuition whispers, "I should check the mailbox today." Experience and pattern recognition say that the metal box on the post near the sidewalk holds letters, and letters are delivered six days a week by a person in a blue uniform; intellect knows that your birthday is five days away. Intuition says that this is the day to check the mailbox. If your intuition is correct, when you open the mailbox, the birthday card from your grandmother will be there with something special in it for you. You learn to listen to that voice in your head the next time. You learn to feel what it is like when your intuition is correct. Intuition is more like a feeling of soft knowing than something you see or hear or experience with your physical senses. To a certain extent, it is taking pattern recognition to a deeper level.

Just as pattern recognition can be learned from sensation, experience, and doing, intuition can be developed by paying attention to what it feels like when intuition is correct and what happens when you do what it suggests. When the quiet whisper or soft vision is more definite, it feels different than when it is equivocal and fleeting. You learn this over time by what happens when you pay attention to the quiet intuition and what happens when you ignore it.

Feedback is the key to informing your intuition and teaching your brain pattern recognition. When the feedback is quick and definite, learning happens quickly and more easily.

It was like that for me when I was learning to use the frequencies to treat patients with FSM. The feedback was the key. It took five years and 25,000 patient treatments for me to become certain that the frequencies always did exactly (and only) what they were described as doing on the list. Once I was certain that the physical feedback was correct, the frequency response trained the pattern recognition that told me which frequencies to use when a tissue felt a certain way or a patient had certain symptoms.

The physical feedback took the form of feeling the tissues soften almost immediately when I used the correct frequency. The tissue would quickly start to feel like a balloon that has been left on the floor overnight. The body surface under my fingers would subtly fall away from my touch. Learning to pay attention to the softening took me quite a long time. For the first few years, I would stay on a frequency that I thought should work for minutes and ignore the fact that the tissue under my fingers remained firm. Experience had to teach me to pay attention to the sensation of softening. Once I recognized the feedback for what it was, it was easy to learn which symptoms went with which tissues and which pathology frequencies would work with those tissues to reduce the pain, produce the softening, and improve health.

I even came up with a word that sounded like exactly what the tissue did. I described this subtle, profound softening as "smoosh."

Smoosh is what the tissue does in response to the frequencies; it doesn't describe what you're doing to the tissue with your fingers. You're not mashing or smashing the tissue. The tissue being treated "smooshes" only in response to the application of the correct frequency that will neutralize what is wrong with that tissue. The softening is best felt when you're using light pressure and your fingers are just sensing the frequency effect. When FSM was first taught in Germany with simultaneous translation, we found out that there is no German word for "smoosh." The German students and the translator looked totally confused when the word *smoosh* was used to describe this softening. But they brightened and understood immediately when smoosh was translated as "pudding."

In 2012, biophysicist James Oschman, PhD, published a paper in *The Journal of Complementary and Alternative Medicine* describing the neurology and physics of tissue softening titled "Visceral and Somatic Disorders: Tissue Softening with Frequency Specific Microcurrent." The FSM community calls it the "smoosh paper."

Intuition is much more subtle. Intuition can be nurtured, informed, and supported. With FSM, the feedback was less definite and discernment much more difficult to learn. For example, when a patient came in with pain and muscle knots all over his body and a history of exposure to organic chemicals and toxins in his print shop, experience and pattern recognition led me to remember the shoulder knots caused by the pesticides in the pear orchard. But how long should the frequencies be used to treat this patient? Should I treat the muscles or treat the liver to help it process the toxins more effectively? Where should the contacts for the current flow be placed? A dim image appeared in my head of my hand placed over his liver so the current could increase the amount of energy available to the liver cells, so I did that. Then, as I thought about how long to treat him, I felt nervous or tight when the idea of anything longer than twenty minutes floated through my mind. Intuition seems to work more on a feeling of relaxation and comfort, of ease and flow, than it does on anything like firm sensation.

LEARNING TO LISTEN

Once I found out how important intuition was to finding the correct treatment, I started paying attention to that feeling of relaxation and ease in all sorts of situations.

Learning to listen to the quiet voice or see the soft images in my head wasn't always easy or painless, and what I learned often came as a surprise. The quiet voice seemed like a puppet at my shoulder repeating advice or replaying particular images until I paid attention to and acted on it. But, at the same time, the quiet voice could be easily overridden by enthusiasm, ego, or wishful thinking.

How do you find the quiet certainty? How do you train it? How do you learn how to feel for it? It is by tuning in to informed intuition, and it will change your life and the lives of those around you.

When we're using frequencies, that training happens every day. The puppet voice at your shoulder suggesting the correct resonant choice is your trainer. You listen and choose and learn to feel what it's like when the voice is correct. You learn discernment and what it feels like when the choice is wrong. You feel it and learn from it hundreds of times every day.

In daily life outside the clinic, the training is less consistent and more subtle. The puppet might send you an image of your favorite aunt. Instead of ignoring the image, call your aunt just to say "Hi." Learn what it feels like when it turns out that she really needed you to call. Slow down enough that you can feel the urge to turn right at the stoplight and pull into a store you haven't visited for years to find the perfect item to fill a need (sweater, vase, kitchen appliance, child's toy, whatever). Learn what it feels like when intuition is correct. And learn what it feels like when it's just a store selling nothing special, and your aunt is fine. That image isn't going to be right all the time. It feels different when it's not tuned perfectly.

That's how you train your intuition. Say yes. Don't bet the farm, but say yes to the soft image inside often enough that you learn what it feels like when it's right and leads you to a better choice. Quiet certainty will follow.

That's how you inform your intuition. You practice and listen to the quiet urgings of your inner voice, feel for the ease, and discover the sense of everything being "right." Follow your passion and put feet on your dreams, even if those feet are wearing baby shoes. Not every step will be a giant step. You can share your truth and still be prudent. You can say yes to the small urges of intuition that guide you along the path and still go to work every day and get the laundry done.

Intuition, even informed intuition, is completely compatible with reason and logical understanding. Someone once told me that I operate almost entirely on intuition and then, in order to teach people how to make that same correct intuitive choice, I reverse engineer it so it seems logical. That might be true, but it doesn't change the process. It's possible that intuition is simply a very refined and subtle form of pattern recognition. Nevertheless, we need to continue learning from all of our senses, even the subtle ones. Seeking information and organizing content to improve pattern recognition is a fairly straightforward process: read books, take workshops, attend lectures, and watch videos. Developing intuition to help with decision-making is a more personal and deliberate process.

If you want to develop your intuition, practice love and gratitude. You attract into your life what you focus on and attract more of what you are grateful for. It's so easy to allow our day-to-day struggles to lock us into dark resentment and disappointment. We have all been there. But it feels like a weight between you and ease. Removing the weight can be a real struggle, or it can be as easy as turning your head.

How do you practice love and gratitude? Make a list of the things you're grateful for that you don't even know you appreciate. Its length will surprise you. Sliced bread. Flush toilets. Clean water. The internet. Gas stations. Cupcakes. Licorice. Vitamin C. Puppies. Horses. Velcro. Dishwashers. Toothbrushes. Kale salad. Cinnamon rolls. Crayons. Erasers. Spackle. Once you get the picture, it's kind of fun. When you make your list, notice how you feel. It feels easy, gentle, and pleasant.

Pleasant positive thoughts become habits of mind by practice, and their use actually changes brain function and even structure in positive ways. It isn't possible to tell yourself, "Don't be irritable and negative." You can't erase a negative with a negative, but it is possible to build a habit of reciting positive words from the list you just made. They might be alphabetical like apricots, bunnies, chocolate, dessert (or even deserts if you like cacti), elephants, fleecy slippers, golf carts—you get the idea. Notice how you feel when you read the list. That feeling of ease and soft comfort is what informed correct intuition feels like.

If you want to develop your intuition, learn to be still inside. The soft urgings of intuition are quiet and easily overpowered by noisy internal dialogue. Practice stopping the internal chatter, and don't yell at yourself. Just be still and silent for a few seconds at a time every day. Formal meditation is a longer version of gazing at a flower for a moment and appreciating its beauty. Most of us just don't have the patience or a schedule that allows us to sit and meditate for an hour at a time, but anyone can be still for a moment and focus on a flower in the sunlight. Intuition means being still to wait for the answer and knowing that it will come when the time is right.

Sometimes we just can't wait for the quiet voice to speak up, and we just do what pops into our head. And sometimes that's when we find out that the quiet voice can just pop into our mind or show up as if in bold print. Sometimes when practitioners are looking at the list and trying to figure out which frequency to use on a problem tissue, one frequency will catch their eye. They can resist the intuition and try to logic their way out of the bold print vision, but intuition can be insistent, tugging on the mind until it responds. The outcome will inform the next choice. Was that frequency correct? Did the tissue go smoosh? Did the frequency reduce the pain?

If you want to develop your intuition, you'll have to get used to making mistakes like a child who has to learn what a hot stove looks and smells like. Doing so is easier when you recognize that there are no mistakes—really. There are outcomes and lessons. It felt like this and you did that, and this is what happened. Outcomes can teach you what to do or not do the next time you have to make a similar choice in response to the subtle urgings of intuition. Intuition takes a long time to develop, and there will be many missteps along the way. Mistakes can make you feel stupid and guilty. But outcomes are just lessons. There is a lesson to be learned from every experience, and there is no profit in resenting experiences that are inconvenient in either impact or timing. *Inconvenient* is a very good word when it comes to providing perspective and nurturing intuition.

Intuition will always bring you what you need. But what you need may not look like what you thought it would look like. Be willing to look for the gift in an unexpected wrapping. Missing that green light may delay your journey, but it might also give you the perfect parking place that would have been occupied if you had arrived three minutes earlier. Learn to be still and say thank you for what is. When the flu puts you in bed, it is never convenient, but sometimes it is the only way you can learn to rest and take care of yourself. When you need your appendix removed and can't get out of bed by yourself, you might learn that it feels good to accept help just this once. And if that help isn't there this time, you might figure out how to get out of bed without using your abdominal muscles and realize how strong you can be when you have to be. The lesson usually becomes apparent only in retrospect. Being grateful for absolutely everything at the time it happens, no matter what it looks like, makes the inevitable lessons a lot more comfortable.

Intuition feels harmonious and soft. When the information around us guides us to a right decision, it feels harmonious. When harmony becomes a habit, it is a lot easier to notice when your intuition is off track and harmony is missing. If you surround yourself with kind, harmonious people and make your living space and actions as harmonious as possible, it feels right, and a lack of harmony is easier to notice.

Find and follow friends who support you and your journey and whose journeys you can support. Do what you are called to do and expect others to do the same for themselves. Everyone will follow their own path for their own reasons. Let them. My mother had a saying, "It has to work for everyone, or it doesn't work." You can learn to choose companions and actions by using the feelings of harmony and ease to guide you. A friend once told me that he was "a student of easy." The school of "easy" always has open enrollment. Pay attention to how you feel when you are with certain people. Do you bring out the best in each other? Even in difficult times of grief or sadness, do you feel better or worse for having been with them? Pay attention to how you feel while you do certain things. Do you feel good? Does it feel easy, as in harmonious? Even when it is difficult or takes effort, does it feel soft and right?

Learning to follow your intuition is not a linear process. Sometimes the puppet on your shoulder is silent—no whisper, no image, no help. Now what? When that happened to me, my intuition decided to teach me how to be methodical about searching for guidance:

The slender, curly-haired thirty-something patient had a simple history. Three years ago, she had gone to the curb, lifted her trash cans into the street for pickup the next day, and hurt her lower back. The pain continued to worsen even when she saw a chiropractor two or three times a week for a year. After that, she said massage made her back worse, so after chiropractic failed to help, she underwent acupuncture. The pain clinic sent her to me when they didn't want to increase her opiate pain medication. The next step for this patient would be an implanted spinal cord stimulator, which everyone wanted to avoid.

Determining the first part of her treatment was easy for me. Massage and acupuncture exacerbated her pain because inflammation in the posterior joints in her spine made it difficult for her to lie on her stomach. She had trigger point knots in her abdominal muscles that referred pain to her lower back. After two weeks of FSM therapy, she was mostly pain-free and able to lie on her stomach. But there was one painful ping-pong ball–sized knot in her lower back muscles that wouldn't melt despite using all of the normal nerve-muscle-joint frequencies.

I listened for the quiet voice. Nothing. Not a whisper. I looked at the frequency list and waited for something to stand out as if in bold print. Nothing stood out to me. Intuition suggested a solution I had never tried before. The painful knot was clearly in the muscle belly, so Channel B was 62 Hz for the muscle belly. Then I went down the Channel A list and tried the pathology frequencies in alphabetical order to see which one would work: A, allergy reaction—no softening; B, the basics—nothing; C, congestion—nope; E, emotional reaction (970 Hz)—the knot softened and the size reduced by half.

What emotional condition could possibly be connected to lifting trash cans? It didn't make sense to me, but since the frequency had worked, I knew it had to be right. But half of a knot remained in her muscle belly, and there was more alphabet left. I tried F, fibrosis—nothing; H, hemorrhage—nothing; I, infection (61 Hz)—the knot disappeared when the muscle softened into smooshy pudding.

Infections? From lifting trash cans?

She propped herself up on her elbow to look at me and exclaimed, "That's it! You did it! It's gone! What was it?"

I replied, "First, let me ask you: what exactly was going on when you lifted those trash cans and hurt your back?"

"That's easy," she said. "My boyfriend and I were splitting up. I had been on the couch with a bad cold for a week, and he was busy moving into his new apartment with his new girlfriend! I was sick and pretty upset. Then, on Sunday, I had to take out the trash because he wasn't there to do it. I grumbled my way to the curb in my fuzzy slippers and bathrobe, jerked the trash cans up off the sidewalk, and zap, my back went out. Why do you ask?"

"I ask because the two frequencies that finished this off were the ones for the emotional component and for a viral infection."

It was hard to tell which of us was more surprised.

Since that experience, when I see a new patient, my intuition makes it a habit of going down the list of pathologies alphabetically in addition to looking for the conditions that make sense to experience and pattern recognition. There are bound to be more surprises.

Be prepared to find out that not every choice will be right and not every lesson will be easy, but every lesson will educate your intellect, improve your pattern recognition, and inform your intuition so that the next choice you make will be closer to right. Be prepared for a stimulating, rewarding, lifelong learning experience in all areas of your life.

Treating patients with frequencies helps with all of this. There are frequency protocols to heal the brain, quiet stress, and balance emotions as well as frequency protocols to repair injuries and improve health. FSM practitioners can treat themselves as well as their patients, and both can improve.

Changing a life by combining education, experience, pattern recognition, and intuition to choose the right frequency and treatment protocol to, for example, eliminate twenty years of chronic pain in a patient makes the whole journey worthwhile.

Carolyn has done a wonderful job of weaving together the practice of FSM and intuition. Modestly, she has not brought forth the profound value of this device for a wide array of medical conditions, so I would like to take a moment to expand on that now.

In addition to the elucidation of cervical trauma fibromyalgia, with which I introduced this chapter, FSM can affect virtually any organ system, and therefore it can be of value for virtually any medical condition. We have frequencies for every area of the brain, every section of the intestines, and every endocrine gland, organ, and tissue. So no matter what is damaged, inflamed, scarred, broken, or torn, we can apply that physiological need to the organ(s) in question.

In my clinic, we have used FSM to help detoxify our sickest patients, reboot the inflamed parts of their brains (especially the vagus nerve for patients with mold toxicity, Lyme disease, or traumatic brain injury), remove the effects of anesthesia that linger years after surgery, help with psychological traumas, and improve the body's ability to make neurotransmitters. We are just beginning to appreciate the applications of this versatile tool. Carolyn has helped us understand that these unique and specific frequencies can be used in the service of both diagnosis and treatment.

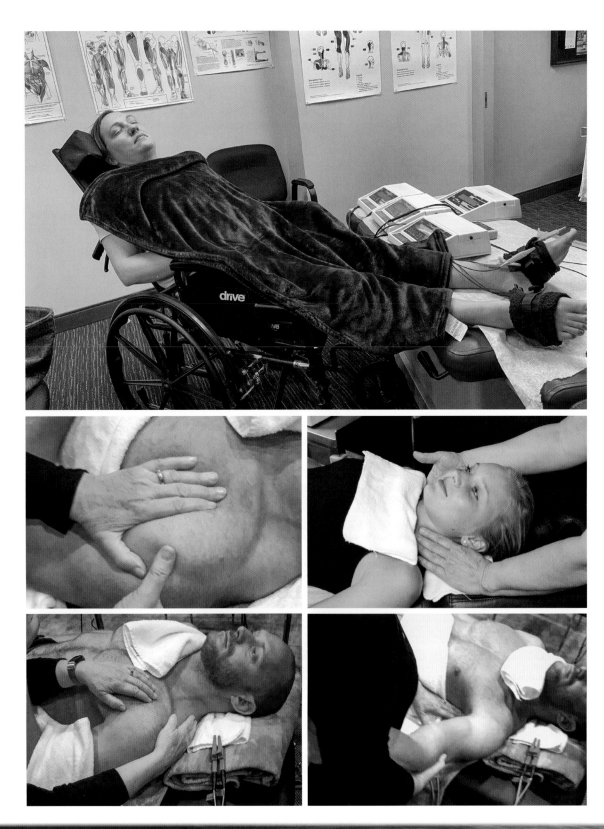

The patient in the top photo is receiving an FSM treatment from the device, which is on the table. You can clearly see the electrodes on her feet; the other pair of electrodes are on the back of her neck (covered by a towel) so that the current is moving from her neck down to her feet, essentially going through her entire body.

The other photos show the placement of the electrodes in treating shoulder pain. The electrodes behind the neck and across the shoulder are conducting the current through those areas. The lower right photo shows how to feel the "smoosh" with the electrodes in place. The hands will feel the softening of tissues when the correct types of current are applied to the patient through Channel A and Channel B concurrently.

Carolyn McMakin, MA, DC, is the clinical director of the Fibromyalgia and Myofascial Pain Clinic of Portland, Oregon. She developed FSM in 1995 and began teaching FSM courses in 1997. In addition to maintaining a part-time clinical practice, she teaches seminars on the use of FSM in the United States, Canada, Australia, Ireland, the UK, Europe, and the Middle East. She has lectured at the National Institutes of Health and at medical conferences in the US, England, Ireland, and Australia on the subjects of fibromyalgia and myofascial pain syndrome, fibromyalgia associated with cervical spine trauma, and on the differential diagnosis and treatment of pain and pain syndromes and sports injuries.

Her peer-reviewed publications include papers on FSM-induced changes in inflammatory cytokines and substance P seen with FSM treatment of fibromyalgia associated with spine trauma, treatment of pain in the head, neck, and face, and lower back pain caused by myofascial trigger points, delayed onset muscle soreness, shingles, and neuropathic pain. She consults with various NFL and MLB teams and players on the use of FSM in the treatment of sports injuries. Her textbook *Frequency Specific Microcurrent in Pain Management* was published in 2010. *The Resonance Effect*, published in March 2017, describes how FSM was developed and provides case reports and frequency protocols for its visceral uses. You can sign up for an FSM seminar, watch FSM videos and webinars, and find frequently asked questions and all of the published and unpublished papers on FSM at www.frequencyspecific.com.

CHAPTER 9:

Muscle Tension Biofeedback, Autonomic Response Testing (A.R.T.), and Intuition

I have had the privilege of knowing and working with Dave Ou for several years. He is one of the contributing authors to my previous book, Toxic, and I was delighted when he agreed to share his unique experience for this book. Here is his story.

by DAVE OU, MD

When Dr. Nathan first invited me to contribute to his book, I did not consider myself to be an intuitive person. I've always thought of myself as a very analytical person with a love of science and mathematics. Prior to medical school, I earned my degree in physics at Cornell University in Ithaca, New York. Before I decided to go into medicine, I had considered becoming an engineer or a computer scientist. I loved the precision of mathematics, and I found that learning physics came more easily for me than it did for most other students. I agreed with the quote attributed to Earnest Rutherford: "Physics is the only real science. The rest are just stamp collecting." I found that biology, which most premed students study, involved primarily memorization and not a lot of thinking compared to physics.

At the same time, I recognized that some of the greatest scientific discoveries, such as Newton's observation of an apple falling from a tree, were attributed to intuition. Einstein said:

> The intellect has little to do on the road to discovery. There comes a leap in consciousness, call it Intuition or what you will, the solution comes to you, and you don't know how or why.

It's hard to explain, but when learning new physics equations, I would try to "feel" what they meant, to give them "life," while it seemed that most everyone else simply memorized them. When solving physics problems, I would try to "feel" the questions, and the answers would usually pop into my head. I would then demonstrate with a series of equations. I never understood how that happened, but, looking back, I used a dance between logic and intuition extensively in my study of physics. This is the way I've always tried to find answers to questions, including in the practice of medicine. Little did I realize that it was the beginning of the road to developing my intuitive skills.

In this chapter, I will describe why I became interested in energy diagnosis, my struggles with learning energy diagnosis, how it has brought joy to my practice of medicine, and some of the lessons I have learned.

EARLY STRUGGLES WITH ENERGY DIAGNOSIS

Since childhood, I have been curious about many things, including the causes of illness. This was largely driven by my own issues with asthma, eczema, insomnia, autoimmunity, and digestive problems as well as my father's health challenges. There are no conventional tests to explain the roots of my health challenges. Much is known about the pathophysiology, and there are many treatments to control, but not cure, the symptoms. I had hoped that there was some other way to determine the roots of my chronic conditions. Given that both my parents were acupuncturists, I knew that practitioners of traditional Chinese medicine (TCM) used pulse and tongue diagnosis (which are components of a comprehensive acupuncture evaluation) to understand the cause of illness. Looking at the tongue in terms of its color, texture, coating, and shape can give us a great deal of information about a patient's overall health. Pulse diagnosis will be covered in greater detail in Chapter 12. This was an important clue that other ways of determining the cause of illness existed.

In college, I read one of Deepak Chopra's books in which he describes how masters of Ayurvedic medicine could make accurate diagnoses with pulse diagnosis. I found it curious that another system of medicine also used pulse diagnosis. At the time, an

Ayurvedic doctor associated with Chopra was scheduled to visit Ithaca, and I wanted to have him analyze my pulse. However, I was disappointed when he ended up having to cancel his plans. My curiosity went unsated until I later consulted a medical doctor trained in Ayurvedic pulse diagnosis. I hoped that through the use of pulse diagnosis, he would find the roots of my illnesses and resolve them. I followed his treatment recommendations, but they had no effect on my symptoms. (As an aside, he eventually became a world-renowned integrative physician and a *New York Times* bestselling author.)

I later consulted several TCM practitioners in the US, China, and Taiwan who used pulse and tongue diagnosis. Each one proclaimed what was out of balance in my body and prescribed herbal cocktails to bring me back into balance, but none of them was able to improve my symptoms.

During medical school and residency, I didn't think too much about energy diagnosis. After my residency in internal medicine, I went into private practice thinking that I would probably get my license in acupuncture if what I had learned in medical school and residency wasn't enough to help my patients. At the time, I thought that Western medical science had all of the answers. I quickly realized the limitations of conventional medicine for many conditions. As a result, I completed the requirements to practice acupuncture in the state of Georgia by taking an acupuncture course for medical doctors to supplement my previous acupuncture training from teachers in China and my parents.

One year, I attended the annual meeting of the American Academy of Medical Acupuncture (AAMA), an organization for medical doctors who practice acupuncture. A class about how to use energetic diagnosis to treat fibromyalgia got my attention because I had found that acupuncture in conjunction with conventional medicine did not seem effective enough for my fibromyalgia patients.

The presenting physician talked about how he used a different style of pulse diagnosis called vascular autonomic signal (VAS), as developed by French neurologist Paul Nogier, to determine which acupuncture points and herbs to use. During the class, he asked for ten volunteers with back pain. By analyzing the pulse of each volunteer, he found a single acupuncture point in each volunteer and placed one needle into an ear. When the volunteers were asked how their back pain was afterward, nine out of ten said that they felt much improved.

I was impressed, and this experience confirmed for me the possibility that energy diagnosis could answer questions and find solutions that conventional medicine could not. I felt it was necessary to have such a tool at my own disposal and wanted to learn how to use it so I could determine which acupoints or treatment a patient needed. Without an energy diagnosis tool, I had to use trial and error of many possible acupoint prescriptions. For back pain, for example, I could try protocol A, protocol B, or Dr. Z's super back protocol. It would be ideal to have a tool to narrow down the best choices.

I don't know why I didn't take a course in the VAS technique. Looking back, I see that my intuition was directing me elsewhere. I first thought about learning what Dietrich Klinghardt, MD (whom I'll come back to shortly), calls muscle tension biofeedback, which is commonly known as muscle testing, but I read that it wasn't always accurate. I later read a physician's website that said non-force kinesiology or leg length testing might be more effective. The general idea of most energy diagnosis systems is to measure the body's response to stimuli; it is similar to a lie detector test in which an interrogator measures pulse, blood pressure, perspiration, and other parameters in response to answers to questions. In this system, the lengths of the legs would appear to change in response to stimuli. The interpretation of the test depends on whether the legs appear to be even or uneven, which would be assessed by placing the thumbs on the ankles and judging symmetry.

I began training with a doctor who taught leg length testing. Curiously, he said that with experience, a practitioner could feel a change in energy before checking for a difference in leg length. At the time, I thought it would be great to have that ability. I tried for a few years to learn leg length testing and feeling for the energy changes, but I couldn't consistently get accurate results. I also became a patient of the leg length testing doctor, hoping he would find the underlying causes of my issues. I did see some improvements, but I hit a treatment plateau and felt something was missing. Years later, I took a class that involved leg length testing, and once again, I could not get it to work. For some reason, it is not the energy diagnosis tool for me.

Undeterred in my desire to learn an energy diagnostic tool, I took a class on testing with a pendulum. I did so partly because my teacher of leg length testing sometimes used a pendulum. The pendulum testing instructor said that to get accurate readings, we needed to do exercises to focus our mind and intuition. However, even after months of practicing, my pendulum seemed to swing randomly. Of course, I had the instructor try to figure out my chronic health conditions, but I had no luck with him, either.

I also tried to learn to use a tool called a Lechner antenna because another medical doctor said that he used it with great success in treating complex illnesses, but I couldn't get it to work. I also consulted a few different medical intuitives who had written books about how they could sense the root causes of a person's illness, but again, I did not have any luck with them.

My next attempt was to try machines that supposedly could read a person's energy. I thought that maybe I wasn't cut out to be an energy tester, and it might be better to let a machine do the work for me. I spent tens of thousands of dollars on various machines, but none of them seemed to be accurate. For one thing, if I ran the test twice, I'd get completely different results. Some of these devices also did energetic treatments, but I did not see much of a therapeutic effect on my patients.

I then decided to learn Electroacupuncture According to Voll (EAV) based on positive reports from medical doctors I knew. With this technique, one uses a probe to measure the electrical resistance at various acupuncture points. Abnormal resistance gives diagnostic information. Any treatment that corrected the abnormal electrical resistance would be considered good. I thought that measuring electrical resistance seemed pretty objective and shouldn't be hard to learn. I took some courses and found EAV to be much harder to pick up than I expected. Each time I would retest the same point, I seemed to get a different reading. The angle of the probe, the degree of pressure, and moisture on the probe could drastically change the reading. For some reason, experienced practitioners would get consistent readings, but I was unable to do so.

Despite my frustrations in learning an energy diagnostic tool and limited improvements in health from such tools, something told me that there was a tool out there that could give me the answers I was seeking. Conventional and functional medical testing could give me some answers, but they were not enough to help many of my complex cases.

LEARNING AUTONOMIC RESPONSE TESTING AND ASSESSING ITS ACCURACY

I ultimately decided to take classes on Autonomic Response Testing (A.R.T.) as developed by Dietrich Klinghardt, MD, and Louisa Williams, DC, ND. Dr. Klinghardt is a world-renowned integrative medical doctor who is especially known for the management of heavy metals and chronic Lyme disease. His energy diagnosis tool of choice is A.R.T. In a nutshell, Drs. Klinghardt and Williams took applied kinesiology (AK) as developed by George Goodheart, DC, and made improvements to reduce false negatives and positives. In AK, or what is known as straight-arm testing, the tester pushes on the patient's arm to see whether they can move it or not in response to pressure. If the arm does not move, it is considered strong, or "good." If it moves, it is considered weak, or "bad." Then the patient is given a vial to hold to see if the contents of the vial improve the response.

For example, a person with a vitamin D deficiency should have a strong arm while holding a vial of vitamin D. However, Drs. Klinghardt and Williams realized that this interpretation is not always true. For example, in many situations, the vitamin D will cause a weak arm in a vitamin D–deficient person. The doctors developed techniques to more accurately interpret arm strength.

A.R.T. also incorporates bi-digital O-ring testing (BDORT) as developed by Yoshiaki Omura, MD, ScD. Dr. Klinghardt added this patented technique to A.R.T. to give additional useful information that cannot be obtained with straight-arm testing. In this technique, the muscles of the fingers are used instead of the arm.

Another feature unique to A.R.T. is the assessment of a concept called biophoton coherence. It is based on the work of German physicist Fritz Albert-Popp, who found that cells and tissues emit light, which is termed *biophotons*. If the cells and tissues are healthy, the biophotons are called coherent. *Coherence* is a term used in physics to describe light that is highly organized, like the light found in lasers. Unhealthy cells or tissues emit light that is described as chaotic and disorganized, called *noncoherent biophotons*. According to Dr. Klinghardt, straight-arm testing can give inaccurate information when biophoton coherence is not taken into account. When a stimulus causes biophoton noncoherence, the arm stays strong no matter what. Remember that in AK, a strong arm is good. However, in A.R.T., a strong arm caused by biophoton noncoherence is not good.

To illustrate, let's look at the assessment of food sensitivities. In a person with a significant gluten sensitivity, gluten causes biophoton incoherence, which causes a strong arm. An A.R.T. practitioner would advise this person to stay away from gluten. A regular muscle tester might say that gluten is good for this person. There is, in fact, a published study comparing A.R.T. with IgE blood testing for food allergies, and it showed a high correlation.

After my first A.R.T. class, I struggled to get the system to work in my office. I took a second class, and I could do the technique successfully during the class. However, when I returned to my office, I still could not get it to work consistently. Refusing to give up, I signed up for another class, but this time, I brought my friend Terry Thompson Horn, MA, who is very intuitive. I knew that she would learn the technique quickly, and she did. Back in my office, I practiced A.R.T. with her, and soon A.R.T. was working for me! People with high levels of intuition like Terry can sometimes transfer some of their skills to other people. I finally had a system that I could use consistently.

Since my goal in learning A.R.T. was to obtain useful information that I could not get with conventional testing, the next step was to verify the accuracy of the information I was getting. It's critical that any test I run, whether it's a lab test, an X-ray, or A.R.T., is accurate. It's important to know or at least consider when a test might be inaccurate.

Let's start with lab testing, which many people mistakenly believe is foolproof. All doctors have seen the results of lab tests that they suspect are faulty because they do not match the clinical picture. Good physicians do not rely 100 percent on test results to guide their assessment and treatment plans. If an abnormal lab or X-ray does not make sense, the doctor will reorder the test, and frequently, the abnormality is not found on the repeat test.

I once had a patient come in with a stack of labs, and she was alarmed that one showed she had mycoplasma pneumonia. She demanded to be treated with antibiotics. However, she did not appear to have any of the typical symptoms, such as fatigue, coughing, or shortness of breath. According to A.R.T., she did not have mycoplasma pneumonia. When I reviewed her labs, I noticed that two different doctors had run a mycoplasma test at the same lab on two different days. One day it was abnormal, and the next day it was normal. For some reason, the result of the first test was wrong, and no one had told her the result of the second test.

Another example of often inaccurate lab testing is food sensitivity testing. I have heard some colleagues say that the accuracy of testing for food sensitivities at various specialty labs is as low as 50 to 60 percent. If you take the same person and send their blood to different labs that specialize in food sensitivity testing, the results from each lab will be different. How can those differences be reconciled? One way is for the patient to try an elimination diet. Another way is through using A.R.T. I once had a patient whose food sensitivity testing showed no reactivity to milk. She started to drink lots of raw milk because she had heard it was healthy to do so. However, she developed fatigue and gastrointestinal symptoms. A.R.T. showed a sensitivity to raw milk, so I advised her to stop consuming it, and her symptoms resolved.

Over the years, A.R.T. has demonstrated consistency with the clinical picture the vast majority of the time. For example, in a patient with low iron or low vitamin D, iron or vitamin D supplements should show good test correlation, and they do. If a patient has cancer in certain organs, I should be able to find it with A.R.T., and I do. I have found that in most anxious patients, A.R.T. shows a benefit from benzodiazepines (medications commonly used to treat anxiety). In most patients with significant pain, A.R.T. reveals the location of the pain and often a benefit from opioids or NSAIDs. In patients with sinus allergies, A.R.T. shows stress in the sinuses and a benefit from antihistamines. In patients with urinary tract infections, A.R.T. shows stress in the bladder and a benefit from antibiotics. If a patient feels a benefit from a particular medication, A.R.T. verifies a benefit the vast majority of the time.

I have been fortunate to have another way to assess the accuracy of A.R.T.: my intuitive friend and colleague, Terry. It turns out that she can feel the effects of treatments, such as supplements or herbs, on people. If a treatment is balancing or supportive, she feels a pleasant sensation. If not, she feels an unpleasant sensation. We have found that there is a strong correlation between what she feels and what A.R.T. shows. If there is a discrepancy, she refines her interpretation of what she feels, or I refine my A.R.T. technique. Through collaborating, we have developed numerous refinements in her intuition and my A.R.T. technique.

One of Terry's skills that helped me to refine my technique is her ability to detect biophoton noncoherence by holding her hands over an organ or tissue. She is able to find such areas that are undetectable with regular A.R.T. I then try to figure out how to refine A.R.T. in order to increase its sensitivity. This has led to breakthroughs in patients whose progress had plateaued.

Through correlation with the clinical picture, laboratory results, and Terry's energetic perceptions, I have gained great confidence in the results of my modified version of A.R.T. However, in the same way that I understand labs aren't 100 percent correct, I keep in mind that A.R.T. isn't 100 percent correct, either, and I always match the results to the clinical picture. The goal of A.R.T. is to be as accurate as possible and to adhere to common sense in all situations.

MINIMIZING GUESSWORK WITH A.R.T.

Once I became comfortable with the accuracy of A.R.T., I wanted to find out if I could use it to achieve my original goal of energy diagnosis, which is to obtain practical information beyond conventional and functional testing. For me, the answer is a definite "yes," and because of this, it has brought joy to my practice of medicine. I act as a detective combining the logic of medical science and access to intuition using A.R.T. to solve medical mysteries that others have not succeeded in solving. Other practitioners of A.R.T. often use the word *fun* when describing their sessions.

Many people do not know that the practice of medicine involves a lot of trial and error. Each symptom can be caused by multiple possible conditions, and each condition has multiple possible treatments and side effects. Healthcare practitioners are always making educated guesses as to what condition a patient has and what treatment will resolve it. If the patient's health doesn't improve, the practitioner makes a different guess and tries another diagnosis and/or treatment. This aspect of medicine was very frustrating for me, and the use of A.R.T. greatly reduces the frustration.

I commonly see patients who develop bronchitis or sinusitis. They initially visit their primary care provider, who makes an educated guess and tells them it's a virus or bacteria. If it is a bacteria, the doctor makes another educated guess as to which antibiotic to prescribe. There is no conventional test outside of a flu test to distinguish among the possibilities, and there is no quick test to help choose the best antibiotic. Most patients recover, but there are always a few who continue to have symptoms. These patients return to their regular physician or perhaps are referred to an ENT or pulmonary specialist, and usually are given another antibiotic based on educated guessing. With A.R.T., I can quickly determine whether the symptoms are due to a virus, a bacteria, an allergy, or some other condition and then determine the combination of antimicrobials or allergy treatments that will resolve the symptoms. A.R.T. minimizes the guesswork and frustration and streamlines the diagnosis and treatment to help patients recover faster.

Another example of the practicality of using A.R.T. to get information beyond conventional testing is locating mercury amalgams under metal crowns in those who are mercury sensitive. It is impossible for a dentist to determine with an X-ray whether a mercury amalgam is present under a metal crown because the metal blocks the X-rays from reaching the amalgam. If dental records are not available, the only way for the dentist to know is to remove the crown. This is an expensive procedure, and no one wants to spend money removing a good crown only to find that there is no mercury underneath. In just about every case in which I have detected an amalgam under a metal crown causing stress in a patient, it has been found when the dentist removed the crown. Using A.R.T. can help streamline dental treatment, saving time and money.

My practice focuses on patients with complex, chronic illnesses who have seen numerous other conventional, complementary, and alternative practitioners without success. Some have even consulted practitioners with whom I have trained. These patients have spent thousands of dollars on labs and treatments. Many have been diagnosed with conditions such as chronic Lyme disease, mold illness, viruses, parasites, heavy metal toxicity, and autoimmunity. Some have been told that it is all in their head. Some have received no diagnosis at all. Many of these conditions are not widely accepted by conventional medicine, and there are few, if any, consensus guidelines on how to approach them.

Before I learned A.R.T., trying to figure out where to begin in these complex cases was very challenging as well as frustrating for me. With A.R.T., I can determine the main issues to address first. Sometimes I discover that an illness found in one of the labs, such as chronic Lyme disease, was not adequately treated. In many other cases, the main issue, such as mold or dental amalgams, was never considered, or a lab returned a false negative. Frequently, many of the positive findings on a patient's lab work, such as a virus or hormone abnormality, contributed to their symptoms in only a minor way, so treating those findings had minimal effect. Through the use of A.R.T., I can identify the major issues and finally help these patients recover.

Another feature of A.R.T. that reduces guesswork and streamlines management is to find treatments that should have a clinical impact and be well tolerated. There are specific A.R.T. techniques that assess what the body's response to a supplement or medication will be. Treatments can have a positive healing response, a neutral response, or a stressful negative response. Other A.R.T. techniques can assess whether a treatment will have an impact on the primary finding, such as an infection or toxin. For example, in a patient with a viral infection, I might find that a probiotic generates a healing response, but it will have no impact on the infection. I might find a supplement that helps with the viral infection, but it causes stress on the body, which would make the patient feel worse. In that case, I would search for a different antiviral. Being able to assess the outcome of a treatment with A.R.T. before recommending it prevents the frustrations of the trial-and-error process that is typically used without the aid of such a technique.

Patients who have had a negative response to nearly every supplement or medication they have ever taken are extra challenging. Without a tool like A.R.T., practitioners aren't sure what to recommend, and patients become frustrated quickly. Trying to find tolerable treatments for these patients is a true test of any energy diagnosis technique. Fortunately, with A.R.T., most of these patients are quite surprised to find that they tolerate my recommendations well, despite their fears. However, I have seen cases in which A.R.T. indicates that a supplement should be well tolerated, but the patient reports that it causes adverse symptoms. When there is a mismatch between A.R.T. and the clinical picture, I try to figure out why, and that has led me to develop new techniques to identify these potential reactions before they occur. This is another example of the dance between logic and intuition.

Another frustrating situation for both practitioners and patients is new or worsening symptoms. Clinicians have to ask themselves whether they are due to a new problem unrelated to treatment, a side effect from treatment, or a worsening of the original problem due to ineffective treatment. There are no conventional tests for this, so the clinician has to make an educated guess and see how the patient responds. With A.R.T., the reason can usually be identified quickly. For example, there was a period when I had started prescribing a new treatment, and over the next couple of months, several hypothyroid patients started to report anxiety, irritability, hot flashes, palpitations, and insomnia, which were unusual symptoms for them. I worried that the new treatment was causing side effects, but A.R.T. indicated that these patients were starting to become hyperthyroid. It turns out that the new treatment was correcting the function of their thyroid gland, so the dose of thyroid medication that they were on became too high for their needs. Lab testing of their thyroid levels along with improvement of their symptoms after decreasing the dose demonstrated that the A.R.T. assessment was correct.

Another use of A.R.T. for which there are no tests is to compare potential treatments. An infection, for instance, can be treated with pharmaceuticals, herbs, homeopathics, and energetic modalities. In the beginning, I wasn't sure if herbs or homeopathics could work as well as or better than pharmaceuticals, but using A.R.T. to determine when they would work better and seeing the clinical improvements after I followed that path has made me a believer. Even though I prefer natural remedies, if pharmaceuticals are the best option, then I will recommend pharmaceuticals. Whenever I learn of a new supplement or modality from a conference, a colleague, or internet research, I can compare it to what I already use. That way, I can sort out marketing hype from reality.

For example, I recently learned the CranioBiotic Technique (CBT), which is supposed to help the body deal with infections, usually chronic, without antibiotics or supplements. The technique involves touching a series of reflex points. As an acupuncturist, I know that acupuncture is generally not useful for the treatment of infections, so I was skeptical that touching certain points could be effective. However, A.R.T. showed that in most cases, the technique would work at least as well as any drug or supplement, and the patients improved. There were still some cases in which antimicrobials were needed, and it's invaluable to have A.R.T. to identify those cases. Through this process of comparing treatments, I am able to upgrade my treatment tools over time.

PITFALLS AND LIMITATIONS OF ENERGY TESTING

It's important to understand that not all muscle testing or energy testing systems are the same. A.R.T. was developed to minimize the inaccuracies of the older testing systems that most muscle testers use. I have made further refinements to A.R.T. to increase its accuracy. It's not uncommon for me to see a new patient who is on dozens of supplements based on muscle testing. Using A.R.T., I find that 95 percent of those supplements are stressing the patient's body and interfering with healing. After I ask the patient to stop taking those supplements, they usually feel better.

One patient, for example, came to see me for digestive symptoms. She had been to a chiropractor for back problems, and the chiropractor said he could do muscle testing to identify the source of her digestive symptoms as well. The chiropractor determined that parasites were the cause and recommended antiparasitic supplements. After taking the supplements, the patient's digestion worsened. When I evaluated the patient with A.R.T., I found that those supplements were aggravating her digestive symptoms. When she stopped taking them, her digestive symptoms improved, and I later treated the root cause of the digestive problems, which was something else entirely.

It's also important to realize that not every practitioner who uses the same good muscle testing system, such as A.R.T., uses it well. I once saw a patient whose health had been getting worse under the care of another A.R.T. practitioner. According to my A.R.T. readings, everything that the previous practitioner tested as "good" was adding stress to the patient's body. I asked the patient to stop taking those supplements, and she experienced immediate improvement. I have seen this happen a few times with patients coming to me from different practitioners. Fortunately, when I see patients managed by other elite A.R.T. practitioners, my readings agree with theirs.

Why do practitioners using the same technique have differing levels of accuracy? There are many possible reasons. One is that A.R.T. practitioners are supposed to make sure that the area in which they perform A.R.T. is free of environmental factors that can cause inaccuracies, such as electromagnetic fields from computers, Wi-Fi, or electrical wiring. I once tried to set up my exam table in a room, but when I checked that part of the room, I detected a stressful factor via A.R.T. Using an electromagnetic field (EMF) meter, I found that there was electrical wiring between the floor of the room and the room below it. After I put some EMF shielding over that part of the floor, I noticed that I got much different results from A.R.T.

The intention of the tester also plays a significant role. A.R.T. practitioners are trained to remain mentally neutral and to push with the exact same amount of force each time. They must not have an emotional attachment to a particular answer. Dr. Klinghardt calls this "honest testing." Many muscle testers will push harder or softer if they consciously or subconsciously lean toward a particular diagnosis or treatment. I once saw a muscle tester who found cancer in everyone. I saw him test twenty people in a row, and he diagnosed all of them with multiple cancers. One could argue that everyone is always developing a small number of malignant cells, but the immune system eliminates those cells. In a way, this practitioner might have been accurate at a microscopic level, but the information was not clinically useful and could be psychologically harmful to patients.

To demonstrate how much intention matters for clear results, a presenter at a conference brought up volunteers to muscle test one another for their response to sugar packets. Most of the time, they tested the sugar packets as "bad." However, it turned out that there was no sugar in the packets, and the volunteers were really testing their beliefs about sugar rather than what was in the packets. The presenter pointed out the effect of intention and beliefs. He also noted that, in reality, sugar might be good for someone who is hypoglycemic but might be bad for a diabetic.

Even A.R.T. practitioners who are technically proficient, maintain neutrality, and perform testing in neutral areas can have different assessments. Most A.R.T. practitioners routinely look for heavy metals, chronic Lyme disease, coinfections, and other infections as the underlying causes of illness. However, many aren't as skilled when it comes to looking for illnesses caused by mycotoxins from water-damaged buildings. The reason is that only some A.R.T. practitioners know to look for mycotoxins and use samples of mycotoxins to test for them. That is no different from a doctor who has not been trained in the diagnosis and management of mold illness. You can't find something if you're not looking for it. This is another example of the dance between logic and intuition.

A common scenario that any practitioner faces, no matter what type of medicine they practice or whether or not they use energy/

intuitive testing, is the persistence of symptoms even though everything that has been identified seems to have been treated adequately. Logically, this means that a known factor hasn't truly been resolved or an unknown factor has yet to be addressed. Just like any lab test, A.R.T. has false negatives. A.R.T. practitioners are always trying to determine how to eliminate false negatives. In other words, how do we find issues that appear to be hiding from A.R.T.?

For example, I recently consulted another practitioner for my own persistent health issues. She found a number of infections and a nickel allergy that I had not previously detected. I asked how she found them, and she showed me her techniques. She demonstrated that A.R.T. will reveal only a limited number of problems at a time. As those problems are sufficiently cleared, A.R.T. can find deeper layers that could not be found before. She finds those hidden layers by treating the current layers during the session. Unlike my previous experiences with energy testing, her recommendations helped me quite a bit. The improvement I've seen in my stubborn health issues has reinforced my belief that the skillful use of A.R.T. can yield very good results.

I view the challenge of restoring health in a chronically ill patient as a series of nested boxes secured by combination locks. To open the first box, one has to determine the exact sequence of numbers. Once the combination is cracked, the next box with another lock is revealed. There are a number of upshots to this approach. The main concept is knowing what to treat and when. A chronically ill patient usually has numerous contributors to their illness, including infections, toxins, interference fields (more on this later), poor detoxification, allergies, and unresolved emotional conflicts. A typical scenario is a patient with chronic Lyme disease living in a moldy home. I usually find that the first combination lock is mold and the second is Lyme. Lyme doctors who are not mold literate will treat the Lyme and wonder why the patient is not getting better. I know it is because they are trying to crack the second lock before unlocking the first. Similarly, a mold-literate doctor who is not Lyme literate will help the patient to some degree by treating for mold but then can't get any more improvements. They successfully cracked the first combination lock but can't open the second. A mold- and Lyme-literate doctor might get past the first two locks and then get stumped by the dozens of locks remaining.

A patient I had previously treated for chronic Lyme disease complained of new foot pain without any history of trauma to that area. With regular A.R.T., I could not find a problem with her foot, nor could I find any Lyme, which I suspected. She had been to a couple of podiatrists who did not find anything wrong. I deduced that for some reason, her body was "hiding" the problem. According to a branch of integrative medicine called homotoxicology, the body sometimes gets tired of fighting an infection or other problem, so it essentially negotiates a truce with the infection and allows it to stay. The immune system effectively reclassifies the infection from high priority to lower priority, like sweeping a problem under the rug.

Science suggests that this could be true. In his Cell Danger Response (CDR) model, Robert Naviaux, MD, says that chronically ill tissues disconnect themselves from central control. It's like closing the bulkheads that separate the compartments in a sinking ship to contain the entry of water. The body can "forget" an infection or diseased area, which makes it invisible to energetic diagnosis.

One way to make the pathology visible is to crack the necessary combination locks. I have been developing new techniques using A.R.T. with the main purpose of finding these hidden or forgotten issues. (More on this later.) In the patient with mysterious foot pain, I went through my process of opening one combination lock after another. Most of the locks were cracked by addressing unresolved emotional conflicts, including feelings of isolation, hopelessness, and grief. I was finally able to detect Lyme and Lyme coinfections in the woman's foot. I treated them, and her foot pain resolved. This process of treating numerous layers before arriving at a previously undetectable deep layer has repeated itself regularly in my practice, so I think it is the norm in chronically ill patients.

INTERFERENCE FIELDS

An important layer that both non-energy-based practitioners and many energy testing practitioners miss is interference fields. One way to describe them is through acupuncture theory. One of the guiding principles in acupuncture is the smooth flow of Qi throughout the body for optimal health. Areas where the flow is blocked can be described as interference fields. In the last century, research on interference fields has found that unhealthy cells have an abnormal resting cell membrane potential. On average, there is a −70 mV difference between the inside and outside of a healthy cell. This is generated by the sodium-potassium pumps in the cell membrane. Dr. Gerald Pollack, author of *The 4th Phase of Water,* would argue that resting cell membrane potential is governed by exclusionary zone (EZ) water surrounding the cell membrane.

Regardless of the explanation, a cell that has an abnormal resting cell membrane potential has difficulty absorbing nutrients and oxygen and excreting toxins. It also is less able to generate ATP, the fuel used by all cells. The most common interference fields are located at scars and in the teeth, sinuses, tonsils, and autonomic ganglia.

The field of integrative medicine that focuses on eliminating interference fields, known as neural therapy, was developed by two German physicians, Walter and Ferdinand Huneke, nearly 100 years ago. In classic neural therapy, interference fields are injected with an anesthetic called procaine, which resets the resting cell membrane potential. In my practice, I sometimes use an energetic device called a LaserCAMS to correct interference fields. In his book, *Neural Therapy: Applied Neurophysiology and Other Topics,* Robert Kidd, MD, writes that CAMS (Crosby Advanced Medical Systems) technology has effectively replaced procaine injections in his practice. When people tell me about medical devices, I tend not to be impressed. I heard about CAMS at an unrelated conference from a random attendee, and for some reason, I was drawn to the technology. Looking back, I suspect it was intuition that convinced me to acquire the device.

Interference fields were also observed in an integrative medical system called Auricular Medicine as developed by Paul Nogier, MD. (Contrary to popular belief, it was Dr. Nogier who discovered ear acupuncture rather than the Chinese.) He created the maps showing which body part each part of the ear is connected to. In Auricular Medicine, interference fields can be treated with ear acupuncture.

I took a class from one of Dr. Nogier's students and learned that interference fields are also common in parts of the brain, including the pineal gland, corpus callosum, cingulate gyrus, hippocampus, thalamus, and hypothalamus. Back in my office, I was able to confirm with A.R.T. that interference fields in the brain are indeed common. It should be noted that I do not know of any way to detect interference fields without some sort of energy testing method, and it is rare that a chronically ill patient does not have any.

INFLUENCE FROM EXTERNAL ENERGIES

Using A.R.T., Dr. Klinghardt has shown that both negative and positive energies can enter the body. At first, this phenomenon seemed very "woo woo" to me, and I wasn't sure it was real. However, over the years, I have found external negative energies impairing the healing process in several of my patients, especially the more treatment-resistant ones. There are many religious, spiritual, supernatural, and New Age explanations for these negative energies, such as curses, attachments, energetic parasites, and entities. I do not know which of these explanations is correct or if it even matters, but they all seem plausible based on my observations. I have several colleagues who are able to sense these energies, and I have started to sense them as well. They appear to drain the energy needed for healing like parasites do.

I have noticed some general patterns in patients who are carrying negative energies. Most importantly, they never seem to have sustained improvement, if they get any improvement at all, even after seeing numerous providers. Some have a "dark" or "negative vibe," while others do not. Dr. Nathan refers to people who are energy vampires in Chapter 6, and most of them seem to have these negative energies. However, only some with the phenomenon are energy vampires. I have found that these negative energies often cause false readings with A.R.T., so I always check for them if my readings do not make sense. I have also noticed that practitioners who carry these negative energies themselves get inaccurate results with their energy testing methods.

In one interesting example, a patient of mine said she was having trouble breathing. A.R.T. showed carbon monoxide poisoning. This did not make sense since the patient didn't smoke or live next to a highway. There were no cars or kerosene heaters in the garage. I decided to run a blood test for carbon monoxide, and to my surprise, it was positive. I performed A.R.T. again. It indicated the presence of an entity who may have died in a fire. I used one of Dr. Klinghardt's techniques to perform a ritual to have the entity leave her body. A.R.T. then showed the carbon monoxide was gone. I repeated the blood test for carbon monoxide, and it had returned to normal.

INTUITION AND SELF-TESTING

Dr. Klinghardt tries to minimize the influence of beliefs and intention in A.R.T. to make it as objective and reproducible as possible. One way he does so is to have practitioners do more "physical testing" than "mental testing." An example of physical testing is using a mercury thermometer to assess mercury toxicity. The mental testing equivalent is to ask the patient to think about mercury or to write the word *mercury* on a piece of paper. Testing with physical objects creates more accurate and consistent results than testing with ideas and concepts. Using physical samples relies more on physiology, while using written words and concepts relies more on intuition, which is more readily distorted by intention and beliefs. Physical testing can be affected by intention and beliefs, too, but it is less prone to those influences. Therefore, A.R.T. practitioners mostly use a collection of glass test vials containing various substances such as medications, herbs, and supplements.

However, I have observed that the practitioners who get the best results when it comes to complex patients appear to be highly intuitive. They just seem to "know" what diagnosis or treatment to look for. In the beginning, I systematically followed an algorithm and would test every vial I had in order to see what issues my patients had and which treatments might help them. This process was time-consuming. The best practitioners cut to the chase by quickly grabbing the vials they think will test positive rather than checking everything. I have asked these practitioners how they do it. One told me that he does self-testing. More specifically, he mentally tests different ideas by using bi-digital O-ring testing of his own fingers. He then confirms his findings with physical testing with A.R.T. The other practitioner said that she just senses what is needed with her intuition and then confirms it physically with A.R.T.

This brings up the question of "who knows" what a patient's response to a stimulus will be. When I first saw the demonstration of using pulse diagnosis to determine the location of an ear acupuncture point at an AAMA conference, the presenter said that everyone in the room should be able to feel a change in their own pulse as the acupuncture point is approached. That means that everyone in the room who is attuned to the patient should be able to sense the patient's energetic status. I have been part of demonstrations with dozens of other students watching Dr. Klinghardt assess a patient. Under the right conditions, if he tests everyone else in the room, each one will test the same way as the patient. For example, if the subject was found to have a weakness in the lungs, everyone in the room would test as having a weakness in their lungs.

This is consistent with my repeated observations that both Terry and my staff members who are present in the testing room often know a patient's response to a test vial even before I put the vial next to the patient. Since the patient's arm is also responsive to the vial, the patient at some level knows the answer as well. Logically, this means that, if trained, we should all be able to determine our own or anyone else's response to a stimulus. It also means that we all should be able to know what is and is not supportive of our bodies if we can only tune into our "knowingness" or intuition. It's just that most people are not in tune with their intuition and need the assistance of another well-trained person to access it.

A few years ago, a patient came into my office with her service dog. The dog appeared hypervigilant, and I was a bit afraid that he might attack my staff or me as we worked on the patient. I was using frequency specific microcurrent (FSM) and dialed into a frequency that A.R.T. indicated was very healing for this patient. My assistant and I both felt a large energy shift. All of a sudden, the dog rolled onto his back and fell asleep. We ran the frequency until A.R.T. indicated that it was done, which took fifteen minutes. The dog stayed asleep during that time. As soon as we turned off the FSM, the dog woke up. Not only that, but he was much friendlier for the rest of the visit. This is a clear example of everyone in the room, including animals, being able to tune into what is going on with the patient.

I agree with Dr. Klinghardt's observation that self-testing, whether it is some sort of muscle testing or the use of a device such as a pendulum, is often less accurate than using another person's muscle, because self-testing is even more prone to beliefs and intention and tends to involve more mental testing than physical testing. For example, I once took a class with a world-renowned muscle tester. I heard that after class, he would use self-testing to decide where to go for dinner, and he would always choose a specific McDonald's. He would then use self-testing to decide what to order, and he always chose Filet-O-Fish, French fries, and Sprite. Since the restaurant had more than one soda fountain, he would self-test and direct the server to get the beverage from a particular fountain. While it is not possible to know for certain whether his self-testing was right or wrong, I was skeptical of the accuracy.

I had tried self-testing with a variety of methods for many years, but it never seemed reliable enough. Since I had struggled for so long to learn energy testing on another person, it makes sense that the most difficult method, self-testing, would be even more challenging. This changed after I worked with two different medical intuitives to help clear some of my emotional and spiritual blocks. Afterward, I attempted self-testing again. I started with checking supplements to see if I needed them or not and then confirmed the results with A.R.T. Once I saw a good correlation, I tried self-testing to anticipate what my patients had and which treatments would be helpful. My self-testing agreed with A.R.T. over 90 percent of the time. I noticed that when there wasn't a correlation, it was always because I was not relaxed or mentally neutral. Just like the previously mentioned A.R.T. practitioners who used intuition or self-testing to more quickly select relevant vials, I became able to do the same. This saves me a lot of time and allows me to address more layers in a shorter period by being able to ask more questions in a shorter period. When pushing someone else's arm, it takes a bit of time for them to prepare their arm before I push and some time before their arm is ready for another push. When pushing my own muscles, there is less preparation and recovery time between pushes.

I learned to self-test after Dr. Nathan asked me to write this chapter. At first, I was just going to write about A.R.T. since I did not think of myself as intuitive. However, after learning about his journey with intuition and then learning to self-test, I looked back at my life and saw how I have been guided by intuition more than I realized. For example, when choosing a supplement with A.R.T., one supplement sometimes stood out in my mind before I even grabbed the vial, and much of the time, A.R.T. confirmed it. Prior to learning to self-test, I would try to ignore those hunches in order to be "objective." I have also noticed that when I listen to a patient, something they say often leads to an idea that pops into my head. This also happens when I am mulling over my patients' problems while lying in bed or driving my car. I now try to pay attention to those ideas. I sometimes call them "intuitive downloads." They remind me of how I used intuition to solve physics problems.

Through the process of paying attention to and trusting my intuition and self-testing, I have explored what I can do with those skills based on what I've heard others can do. One example is to use self-testing to physically locate a remedy for a patient. This is based on a story told by one of my intuitive friends, William McCarthy. He went to a restaurant for dinner and wanted to order a side of coleslaw. The waitress said they were out of coleslaw. While in his booth, he mentally scanned the restaurant with his intuition and then told her to look in the corner of a specific shelf of a secondary refrigerator. She insisted there was no coleslaw to be found, but to humor him, she went to where he told her to look and was surprised to find coleslaw there.

I have numerous boxes containing thousands of sample vials of medications, nutrients, herbs, and homeopathics. If I need to find a remedy for a particular symptom, I sometimes use self-testing, like William does, to narrow down in which part of my office a helpful remedy will be found, then which shelf or drawer, then which box, and then which row and column in the box. Over 80 percent of the time, when I test that sample vial using A.R.T., it tests as very beneficial to the patient. It is not uncommon that I pick a vial I forgot I even had.

If specific items can be found with intuition, it would make sense that acupuncture points and the pathways along which they lie, called meridians, were almost certainly found through intuition thousands of years ago. Similarly, the energy vortexes in Ayurvedic medicine, called chakras, were very likely discovered through intuition. Even though my parents were acupuncturists and I was trained in acupuncture, I was never quite sure that meridians were real until I learned from Dr. Klinghardt how to find them with A.R.T. He also teaches how to find and assess chakras with A.R.T.

I wrote earlier about a technique called CranioBiotics (CBT), in which reflex points for bacterial, viral, fungal, and parasitic infections have been mapped. Intuitively, I wondered if there were reflex points for other clinical issues. For example, I asked if there were reflex points for the detoxification of heavy metals, and my self-testing directed me to an area around the kidneys. I have verified those reflex points with A.R.T. and have found them useful in assisting the body in managing toxic loads. I have found reflex points for infections not taught in CBT, such as *Bartonella, Babesia,* and retroviruses. I have also found reflex points for autoimmunity, as well as airborne, food, and other allergies.

I have discovered the reasons why CBT and other reflex point–based systems are sometimes unsuccessful in clearing chronic infections and allergies, and in the process how false negatives with energy testing can occur. I have noticed on many occasions that patients who had been treated for chronic infections were still having symptoms even though A.R.T. showed that the infections had been cleared. Using intuition and self-testing, I asked if there were reflex points that would reveal that the infections were still there. In other words, could there be reflex points that would unmask these infections? I confirmed those points with A.R.T., and after I treated those reflex points, the chronic infections would show up with A.R.T. again. I would treat the infection again, and it would test as having been cleared, but the patient would still be symptomatic. I would have to intuitively find more reflex points to unmask that the infection persisted. This cycle would continue many times. It was especially common in complex, chronic illnesses such as chronic Lyme disease.

It turns out that the majority of these unmasking points are located on meridians, chakras, and another energy pathway called the hara. Blocks in the meridians, chakras, and hara are traditionally thought to be related to unresolved emotional conflicts. I discussed in an earlier section how the body can "forget" infections and diseased tissues through the Cell Danger Response, making them invisible to energy testing. Addressing emotional blocks through these unmasking points appears to help the body "remember" that infections and disease are still present and in turn make them visible to energy testing. Also, reconnecting these forgotten issues to central control is a crucial component of healing from chronic illness according to the CDR model.

My intuition has led to me revisit energy healing. One way to describe energy healing is using intention to improve energy balance in the body. Better known examples include Reiki, Qigong, and the laying on of hands. I have been certified in a system called Matrix Energetics and have taken classes such as Reconnective

Healing and Body Code. I had not used energy healing much in my practice because the results appeared inconsistent. I always blamed it on my not being intuitive enough. Once I developed more confidence in my intuition, I started to treat reflex points using intention based on my training in energy healing with good results.

All energy healing systems say that when energy is balanced in the body, health is restored. However, I have not found any systems that seem consistent in being able to resolve complex, chronic illnesses. Even in childhood, I always sensed that it would be possible to create such a system. This may be why I always felt a strong need to learn energy testing as a tool to develop my intuition, which was necessary to develop such a system.

At the time of publication, I have not yet finalized this system. What I know so far is that the sequence of treating reflex points is like a combination lock. If the combination is not correct, the body starts to give inaccurate information with energy testing, and the results will be suboptimal. For complex cases, merely treating reflex points for toxins and infections will not yield the best results. It appears that for complex cases, it is important to address unresolved emotional conflicts. My intuition has led me to a principle that exists in nearly all systems of traditional medicine: in order to achieve true healing, the mind, body, and spirit all have to be addressed.

CONCLUSION

My journey to learn energy diagnosis through A.R.T. and to access my own intuition has not been easy. For some reason, since I was young, I knew that I needed access to such tools. These tools have been invaluable in relieving the suffering of those who have been unable to find help from more traditional healthcare modalities. It is gratifying and rewarding to practice medicine with these tools. Now, with my newfound access to intuition, I expect that I will continue to gain new insights into how to optimize health and share those insights with others.

I will conclude with a story of how my new techniques developed through intuition helped a patient who recently returned to my care.

Sherry is a forty-year-old registered nurse who developed fatigue, pain, headaches, anxiety, and constipation in 2008. A few years later, a Lyme-literate medical doctor (LLMD) diagnosed her with chronic Lyme disease. She was given multiple rounds of oral and intravenous antibiotics with no benefit. She also had several rounds of intravenous silver and ozone without benefit. She took numerous supplements under the care of a naturopath with no benefit. By 2015, Sherry was so fatigued that she had to quit nursing. I saw her in 2017 and via A.R.T. found Lyme coinfections, viruses, bacteria, and parasites. I treated those with herbs and then Biomagnetic Pair Therapy as developed by Isaac Goiz Duran, MD. However, she did not see any sustained improvement over a year.

She left my practice for a year to pursue treatments for other issues. She then returned because her pain had gotten worse, she had developed new numbness and tingling, and her fatigue was still significant. Intuitively, I felt there was an external negative energy that kept her from clearing Lyme and the coinfections. With A.R.T., I found an external negative energy along with several associated unresolved emotional conflicts and three Lyme coinfections: chlamydia pneumonia, mycoplasma, and rickettsia. I felt that the main blockage to her healing was the external energy, which I had not looked for in previous visits. I addressed the external energy by using several Bach flower remedies for the associated unresolved emotional conflicts. I treated the Lyme coinfections with my modified version of CBT. I used Soliman Auricular Allergy Treatment (SAAT) to neutralize her neurological intolerance to gluten, milk, and Xanax as well as the antibodies to progesterone, estrogen, Epstein-Barr virus, strep, brain, myelin sheath, and lacrimal glands.

I performed noninvasive neural therapy using a LaserCAMS on interference fields in the brain, sinuses, teeth, thymus gland, small intestine, uterus, esophagus, ovaries, and neck. After doing all that, the bacteria Borrelia was unmasked, which I treated with CBT.

When Sherry returned to my office two months later, she reported that her fatigue, pain, numbness, tingling, brain fog, constipation, and headaches had lessened considerably. She said that this was the best she had felt in years. She had improved so much that she started to look for a job after being unable to work for five years. This is the power of energetic healing: being able to change lives when things look their bleakest. Energetic intuition gives hope to those who felt hopeless.

LaserCAMS device used in the treatment of interference fields.

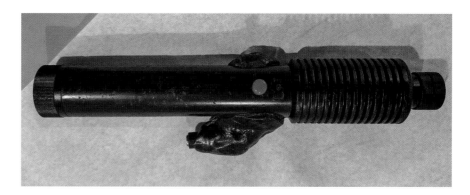

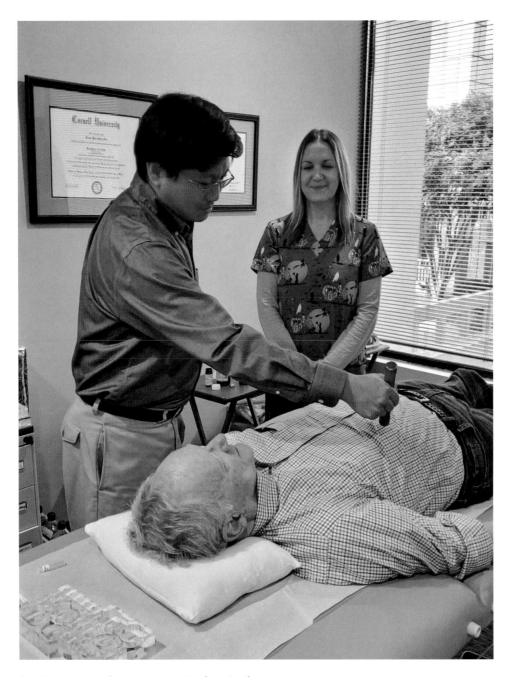

Dr. Ou is using the Lemurian Healing Rod in treating a patient.

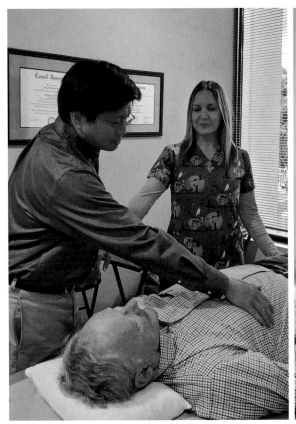

Dr. Ou is using A.R.T. to evaluate a patient's liver.

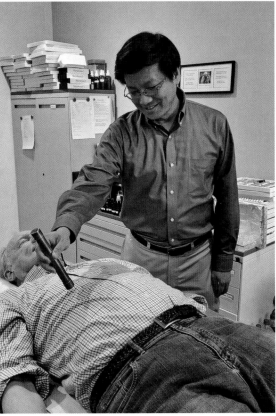

Dr. Ou is using a Lemurian Healing Rod to treat a patient energetically.

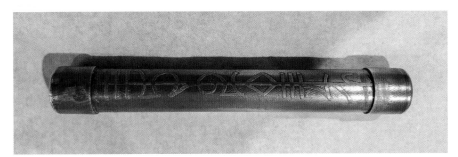

Lemurian Healing Rod.

Dr. Dave W. Ou graduated cum laude from Cornell University with a BA in physics, received his MD from the University of Miami School of Medicine, and completed his residency in internal medicine at Emory University. He has been board certified in internal medicine since 1999. After practicing internal medicine for ten years, he started a private practice in integrative medicine in Atlanta, Georgia, focusing on complex, chronic illnesses primarily through the use of energy medicine. He was certified in Autonomic Response Testing by Dr. Klinghardt in 2014. Learn more at his website, www.bridgestohealthatl.com, and on Facebook at www.facebook.com/bridgestohealthatl.

CHAPTER 10:
Reiki

I had the privilege of working with Sonia Rapaport, MD, several years ago to help orchestrate a medical meeting that was exceptionally well received. Since then, we have worked closely together as friends and colleagues, and I am delighted that she has agreed to share some of her wisdom and experiences with energetic medicine. Here's Sonia.

by SONIA RAPAPORT, MD

There is nothing more frightening than having a sick child, especially when no good treatments are available. My youngest daughter, Sarah, was a few months old when I discovered that she and her older brother, Sam, have a rare genetic disorder called familial dysautonomia (FD). Sarah's nervous system would react wildly to the slightest input, and she would cry inconsolably. Going to synagogue services was impossible that first year. Heightened energy, even the focused energy of the congregation praying, made her scream. With the diagnosis of FD, I discovered that she was experiencing a sympathetic (flight-or-fight) response very quickly. The medical treatment at the time was to calm the nervous system with the use of medications like Valium. I had spent much of my career trying to get patients off addictive drugs like Valium and couldn't imagine my baby living on it.

So when a friend named Sara told me about Reiki, a decades-old form of hands-on healing that had been passed down through generations of energy healers, I was intrigued. I had witnessed the power of touch with my son Sam. When he was an infant, he was hospitalized with a severe respiratory infection. It was before I knew he had FD, and the severity of his condition was unexpected. He was transferred to a major medical center, where he was placed on oxygen. Because Sam couldn't clear the mucus in his lungs, his oxygen would drop to dangerously low levels, and the medical staff was considering putting him on a ventilator, which would breathe for him.

Standing by his crib, I could do little but hold him. I placed my hands on his chest, and as he breathed in and out, I visualized the air entering his lungs and the mucus moving up and out. Each time I did this visualization, Sam's oxygen saturation (oxygen levels) would improve from the low 90s to the mid-90s and stay at the higher level for ten to fifteen minutes. I was pouring all my love and energy into him, and the energy I was expending to visualize and help him mobilize the mucus was exhausting.

When Sara told me that she'd been trained to do Reiki, I knew she would be able to help Sam and Sarah. I witnessed her calm Sarah with a gentle touch. She told me that Reiki uses universal healing energy, rather than the practitioner's personal energy. It was a sustainable form of energy healing. I signed up for the next Reiki class I could find.

Reiki is a form of hands-on energy healing in which a Reiki practitioner begins with the intention of receiving the universal healing energy and then transmits that energy to an individual in need of healing. Reiki, in its basic form, is a natural impulse. We reach out to touch someone who is hurting. Parents kiss and rub their children's boo-boos. Many of us begin to relax at the thought of having a massage. Reiki uses the energy inherent in the universe to heal. A Reiki practitioner taps into that energy, and in the process also receives some of that energy.

HISTORY

Reiki comes from the Japanese words *Rei,* which means "universal life," and *ki,* which means "energy." Reiki was first discovered in Japan by Mikao Usui. Dr. Usui was born in 1865 to a wealthy Japanese family. He was educated at a Buddhist monastery, where he began his study of medicine. During that training, he underwent a three-week solitary retreat in a cave on Mount Kurama. During those twenty-one days, he fasted, prayed, and meditated. On the last day, he was given a vision of ancient Sanskrit symbols that allowed him to develop the healing system he called Reiki. Dr. Usui continued to develop his healing system, and in 1922, he opened a Reiki clinic and school in Tokyo.

After Dr. Usui's death in 1926, one of his students, Chujiro Hayashi, refined the training process for teaching Reiki and expanded the school. It was there, in 1935, that Hawayo Takata, a woman of American-Japanese descent from Hawaii, learned about Reiki. Takata had traveled to Japan to seek treatment for cancer. When her doctor recommended surgery, Takata trusted her instinct that she didn't need surgery to be healed and asked for alternative treatments. She was told about Dr. Hayashi's clinic, and although she was initially skeptical, she sought out his care. Over time, with daily Reiki treatments, she was healed.

Takata was so impressed with the healing she experienced that she petitioned Dr. Hayashi to allow her to study Reiki. In the male-dominated culture of pre-World War II Japan, women had not been permitted entry to Reiki training, but Dr. Hayashi admitted her to the school, and Takata became the first female Reiki Master. After returning home to Hawaii, Takata continued to practice Reiki, and over the years she attuned twenty-two Reiki Masters.

REIKI TRAINING

Reiki is passed to students by a Reiki Master, who has received advanced training and undergone an apprenticeship in Reiki. There are three levels of Reiki training: First Degree, Second Degree (or higher power), and Third Degree (or Reiki Master). In the United States, a Reiki Master's lineage refers to the line of teachers that can be traced back to the first US Reiki Master, Mrs. Takata. The fewer the teachers in a Master's lineage, the closer to Classic Usui Reiki they are thought to be. Reiki doesn't require additional medical training, however—the energy goes where it's needed—so even children can learn to do Reiki.

During basic or First Degree Reiki training, a Reiki Master teaches her students the Reiki method and the Reiki philosophy of healing. After students are properly introduced to these basics, they receive a ritual attunement during which their crown chakra is opened to the universal healing energy. Most Reiki Masters include a hands-on session as part of their class, allowing students to practice the techniques on each other and ensuring that they have properly learned the Reiki positions, or where and how to properly place one's hands on a client.

During Second Degree training, a student learns more about the practice of Reiki, including specific symbols and phrases that are used with clients. Most Reiki Masters ask that a student practice First Degree Reiki for at least six months before advancing to Second Degree. Second Degree Reiki training confers an ability to access Reiki energy at a higher or more potent level, accelerating the healing process. The Reiki symbols and phrases are also used to deliver healing long-distance and for psychological support, helping to refocus the mind on more productive thoughts and emotions. Emotional healing through Reiki is a collaborative process where the Reiki practitioner and client work together to find the best phrases to gently suggest during a session.

Third Degree training confers the title of Reiki Master on a practitioner and is offered to students after at least a year of practice with Second Degree Reiki. A Third Degree Reiki student apprentices with a Reiki Master generally for six to twelve months, helping to teach classes, continuing their own work with clients, and perfecting their practice of self-care and awareness. Reiki Master apprentices learn how to conduct attunements in preparation of teaching Reiki.

REIKI PRACTICE

What healers say makes a difference. How they say it can make even more of a difference. I studied with a Native American medicine man in medical school. "To get someone to respond best to a prescription, tell him to take it under a tree," he told me. Placebo? Belief system? Trust? Or is any therapy energetically more potent when connected to Mother Earth? To universal healing energies? Energy healing, like Reiki, connects all of these dots. The myth of Reiki's discovery is part spiritual journey, part earth connection, part healer's journey, but how Dr. Usui found Reiki isn't what matters to the people who have been healed by it. What matters is its power, which is all about human touch.

After I got my first Reiki attunement, I could calm my daughter Sarah much more easily and thoroughly than was possible before the attunement. Holding her in my arms with my hand on her belly doing Reiki soothed her and helped calm her nervous system. I had seen the impact of my touch when Sam had been hospitalized, but with Reiki, it became much more powerful. I didn't need to expend my own energy to have a positive effect on the people I treated.

My First Degree attunement was from a wonderful healer named Berkely Reynolds, and I immediately wanted to study more. Berkely had strict requirements. Her classes were weekend-long programs, and no one could study for the next level without a minimum of six months of practice at the first level. As soon as I was able, I signed up for Second Degree training, and I signed up my two oldest children, Ben and Rachel, for First Degree Reiki attunements. Ben was seven and Rachel was five years old.

Shortly after we received the training, a friend named Mary fractured both her legs in a car accident. Ben and Rachel were excited to be able to help, and we went to visit her. Because of the swelling of her legs, the orthopedist hadn't casted her legs yet. We offered to do Reiki. As we sat and talked, I placed my hands on one leg, and Ben and Rachel placed their hands on the other. Many Reiki practitioners note warmth or tingling in their hands when they do Reiki, but Rachel's hands would get particularly hot, and she had been taught that heat meant that she was touching a place in need of healing. After ten minutes of Reiki, Rachel complained that her hands were too hot and she took them off Mary's leg.

That evening, Mary called me. Several church members had visited her after we left, and one of them remarked how odd it was that she had an area in the shape of a child's hand on one leg that was less bruised than the surrounding skin. While proper Reiki form involves holding the fingers together, Rachel had spread her fingers on Mary's leg. The Reiki energy had begun to resolve the bruise where Rachel placed her hand.

I was fortunate in those early years of Reiki practice to be part of a thriving healing community with many other Reiki practitioners. We studied together and had regular Reiki circles. At a Reiki circle, practitioners take turns doing Reiki on each other, treating different positions simultaneously. A Reiki circle can also treat someone rapidly. When one of the other practitioners developed a slipped disc, for example, we all gathered to do Reiki on her back, and within an hour she felt significantly better.

But it was Joe's sudden death that brought home the importance of our Reiki circles. The tragedy left his widow, Kim, a single mother with young children, and despite her grief, she had to continue on. It was with Kim that I felt the tremendous power of Second Degree Reiki. There are several positions in which one places their hands when doing a Reiki session, including over the heart. Our Reiki circle gathered for Kim and we began with each of us placing our hands in a different position, but it became clear that the position that was drawing the most energy was Kim's heart. One by one, we stacked our hands on the heart position. Several of us used the higher power of Second Degree Reiki, feeling the heat and tingling rise and fall for nearly an hour. It was the most synergistic Reiki session I've ever participated in; the love that surrounded Kim that day was palpable.

I became a Reiki Master in 2001 and when I opened my medical practice in Chapel Hill six years later, I offered Reiki sessions to patients. One young woman I saw early on in my practice had been sexually abused as a child. She was under the care of a wonderful therapist, who was doing cognitive behavioral therapy with her, but she felt that something was missing in her treatment. While the cognitive behavioral therapy was helping her understand and process what had happened, she felt that the emotional and spiritual component of the abuse was not being adequately addressed. We worked together to improve her recovery in several ways, and we concluded each appointment with a Reiki session, using Third Degree Reiki to address the history of abuse.

With each session, I asked her what she wanted to address. Being the victim of abuse, she was averse to touch, but because she had come to trust me, I was able to place my hands on her head and, through Reiki, provide the flow of healing energy. Reiki was an adjunct to the psychological therapy, and over the course of her treatment, she had significant breakthroughs and healing. What was remarkable for me to witness was that the healing was not coming *from* me, but instead, the energy was flowing *through* me. I was a tool for her body to access and use the universal healing energy that surrounds us. I learned from this brave young woman that healing occurs in the person who needs the healing; I merely helped provide access to the energy that accelerated the process.

Sam and Sarah are young adults now, and they have received Reiki attunements as well. Reiki has been a steady part of their lives, both receiving and giving Reiki energy. Over the course of their lives, Reiki has given me a tool when there were no others, an ability to go beyond my love as a mother and tap into the loving energy that surrounds all of us. There were times when Reiki helped to keep Sarah out of the hospital. I did Reiki to clear the energy of rooms when they were admitted to the hospital. With Reiki I was able to calm Sam as he was having an intravenous catheter (IV) placed when he was hospitalized. Reiki gave me the knowledge that I was not alone in caring for my children. The universe was there to help.

Whether you're a Reiki practitioner, you've had Reiki treatments, or even if you have never heard of Reiki before, the benefits of Reiki healing extend beyond hands-on energy work to help anyone in need of loving energy through Dr. Usui's Reiki Affirmation, which states:

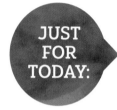

JUST FOR TODAY:

- I WILL NOT WORRY
- I WILL NOT BE ANGRY
- I WILL DO MY WORK HONESTLY
- I WILL GIVE THANKS FOR MY MANY BLESSINGS
- I WILL BE KIND TO MY NEIGHBOR AND ALL LIVING THINGS

Sonia Rapaport, MD, has been treating patients with complex illnesses since 1997. She began her career as a board-certified Family Physician and is certified in Functional Medicine (IFM), Integrative and Holistic Medicine (ABIHM), SCENAR therapy. She has been a Reiki Master since 2001. In 2017, she founded and became the first president of the International Society of Environmentally Acquired Illness (ISEAI). She works with patients who have not improved with conventional treatments and those who are so sensitive that they can't tolerate drugs or even natural products well. Her patients often have complex medical conditions such as mold illness, tick-borne diseases, mast cell activation, dysautonomia, and hypermobility.

Dr. Rapaport has lectured nationally and internationally on environmentally acquired illness, integrative medicine, dysautonomia, and narrative medicine. She holds an MA in medical anthropology, an MFA in creative writing, and is a WTA certified Tea Sommelier, and Tea and Health Expert.

Dr. Rapaport is the founder and director of Haven Medical in North Carolina. Contact her through her website, www.SoniaRapaportMD.com.

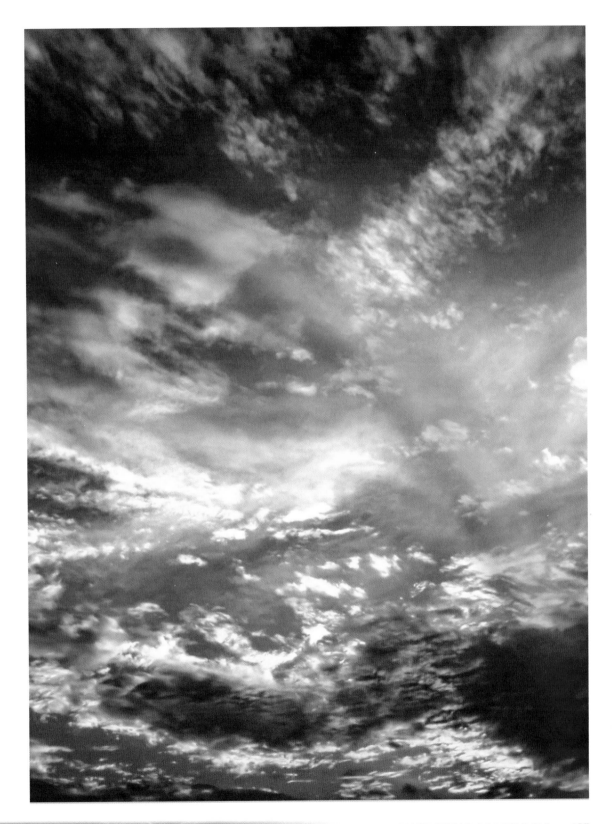

CHAPTER 11:

The Healing Potential of Dowsing and Its Use in Energetic Diagnosis

Later in this chapter, Dr. D alludes to meeting some "medical malcontents" at an American Holistic Medical Association (AHMA) meeting many years ago. What he does not mention is that I was one of them.

At one of these early meetings, in 1982, my good friend Carolyn Torkelson, with whom I was working at the time, came up to me and insisted that I follow her immediately to meet a young physician whom she felt "could be my brother." Intrigued, I was introduced to Dr. D. Here is another example of energetic resonance or recognition: Dr. D and I became immediate friends and were inseparable for the rest of the meeting. We have led remarkably parallel lives: having children of about the same age, getting divorced at the same time, and later finding our loving soul mates. We remain the best of friends.

On my first day of medical school in 1967, I, too, was informed that 50 percent of what I learned would be proven false (but in my memory, it would take twenty years for that to become known to me). Virtually every student in every medical school gets the same orientation, but I took the information a bit differently than Dr. D did, as he will describe momentarily. To me, it meant that I needed to keep an open mind as to what was becoming known to be true, which was clearly a work in progress. It meant that I was embarking on a lifetime of study and learning, and that was fine by me. I love to learn.

As Dr. D correctly observes, most of our classmates did not take in this information as we did. Most physicians are so exhausted from their years of medical school and residency training that they hope what they have learned will last them until retirement. Obviously, it will not. But in my experience, it is rare for physicians to recognize that they must continue to pursue medical knowledge throughout their career. That most do not helps to explain why the practice of medicine is in the sorry state that it is and why patients are so frustrated with many of their treatments. It also helps to explain why the majority of physicians are so slow to embrace new concepts and ideas: it has taken twenty-plus years *for medicine to even begin to accept the epidemic of Lyme disease, although the Centers for Disease Control admits that over 400,000 new cases are identified in the US every year. The epidemic of mold toxicity is even newer and less accepted, despite the estimate that 10 million Americans are suffering with some form of it right now.*

Let me allow Dr. D to get going on his fascinating story, which will light up a number of important areas to understand in the field of energy medicine.

GETTING BEYOND 30 PERCENT

by **DR. D**

To properly understand what needs to be said about sound healing, context must be provided. Whoever said "context is everything" was telling the truth. What I am about to share is personal; there is no other way around it. Personal discovery is not a scientific report, nor should it be mistaken for universal truth.

This story begins in the fall of 1976, on my first day of medical school. All of the new students were assembled in the auditorium that would serve as a second home over the next two years. The dean gave the "Welcome to medical school" lecture, but the incoming class seemed restless, as if to say, "Let's get on with it." For whatever reason, my ears were wide open during his first and only talk with our full class. He said many things during the next hour, but a few stood out to me and actually determined my trajectory for the next forty years.

In attempting to implant in us a sense of gratitude, as if to say, "You are the most fortunate group to be granted entry into this halcyon institution," the dean launched into how great and advanced his medical school had become. All of the schools in the South fancied themselves the Mass General or the Mayo of the South. (At that time, the Mayo Clinic's Florida campus did not exist.) I'm sure the students at Duke, Vanderbilt, and Emory all heard similar opening-day lectures. Regardless of who was indeed the top dog, all suffered from grandiose self-appraisal. The dean then explained just how fast medical science was advancing. The advancement was so fast, in fact, that by the time we graduated in four years, 50 percent of everything we had learned would have been proven wrong. Stunned,

I looked around the room to see if this shocking statement registered on anyone else's face. I saw only blank faces. On the heels of that statement, the dean said that we do not know which 50 percent would be proven incorrect. I thought to myself, "I am going to bust my ass for four years, and in the end, I will have to discard two of those years. Such a deal!"

The dean was not through with his bombshells. He stated that the Mayo Clinic had a 30 percent correct diagnostic and treatment rate and that our medical school was right behind them, as if 30 percent was something to be proud of. I quickly connected the dots. I knew Mayo quality, and most of their doctors were under the far end of the Bell Curve. I have never had the level of intellect of the folks at Mayo, and an honest self-assessment put me under the tall part of the Bell Curve, probably edging closer to the near end. If these very bright doctors were right only 30 percent of the time, what could I hope for? On a good day, maybe 20 to 25 percent?

Mayo had the cream of the crop; it was not for want of intelligence that they had a 30 percent correct diagnostic and treatment rate. So what was the dean telling us? Quite simply, that the science we were about to learn (allopathic medicine) was good and indeed proper for up to 30 percent of what we would encounter, if we turned out to be very bright. The percentage would be lower for those of us who were average. To me, this was wholly unacceptable. Would you leave your car with a mechanic who told you they had a one-in-three chance of properly fixing the car? I wouldn't. What the dean was really saying was that allopathic medicine is an incomplete approach to understanding and treatment. No one else seemed to have heard it in the way I did.

I rapidly concluded that since my MD training was not going to reveal the other 70 percent, it was up to me to find it. The next forty years would be my adventure into that 70 percent. As it turned out, the dean's 30 percent number was remarkably accurate. About a third of my patients receive appropriate allopathic care.

Getting through the next four years required me to give everything I had. It seemed like a stiff price to pay to learn less than one-third of what I would need to know as a doctor. The 70 percent had to wait until after I graduated, but the hard truth that I was exhausting myself to learn a very incomplete system of healing made it difficult to buy into the philosophical underpinnings of allopathy. While I was surrounded by arrogant teachers and classmates, I could not fathom the reason for their arrogance. Even if these self-assured students and physicians were superb, they could help only one in three patients. For the other two-thirds of patients for whom allopathy simply is not effective, failure and often tragedy awaited. Considering this, how could one possibly be arrogant? I fought the unspoken teaching that MD stands for Major Deity. If failing two-thirds of the time does not make one humble, there is something seriously amiss. I am not saying that all doctors are narcissistic or power mad, but if the shoe fits....

For this reason, I have been as humble as my personality will allow. My education started after I got my MD degree; I was (and am) committed to being the best healer (notice I did not say "doctor") I could be, and I set about to discover the unknown 70 percent.

It was not hard to figure out the bulk of this body of knowledge. A number of people, organizations, and alternative therapies played a pivotal role. In the early 1980s, the AHMA meetings were transformational. I found myself surrounded by others like myself— pariahs and allopathic malcontents. I learned about nutrition, self-care, acupuncture, traditional osteopathy (which was nothing like they teach in osteopathic medical schools today), homeopathy, and various psychotherapeutic approaches. At those gatherings, I met many of the future movers and shakers in the alternative medical movement. The presenters at the AHMA meetings represented a wide slice of humanity and doctors working on the edges of allopathic medicine. At various times, these understandings and techniques have been of tremendous value to me.

The central tenet of holistic medicine is that we are composites of three interacting spheres: physical, mental/emotional, and spiritual. For the most part, allopathy addresses only the physical and leaves psychiatrists to deal with the rest. No wonder it is so ineffective; it ignores the spiritual aspects of being altogether and relegates mental health treatment to a drug model or, as American philosopher/psychologist William James referred to it, "medical materialism." The holistic model has served me well and provides a template for me to discern which way to go with any given patient.

Symptoms and disease always have an origin. If all we are interested in is eliminating or abating symptoms, we will never even think to ask about their origin. Each symptom or disease can arise predominantly from either the physical, mental/emotional, or spiritual realm. If I fail to discern the origin, the treatment I provide will be ineffective at best and harmful at worst. Heeding the first Hippocratic injunction to "do no harm" is challenging when one follows a traditional allopathic model. So much harm is done nowadays, and it is easy to see why.

If a symptom has an emotional origin, treating it as having a physical source will produce little if any benefit. The reverse is also true. Treating something purely physical with a psychology-based solution will be no solution at all. In a very real sense, I do my own triage: find out the source of the problem and then devise a therapeutic regimen from that domain. A physical source problem gets a physical solution, a mental/emotional source problem gets a mental/emotional solution, and a spiritual source problem gets a spiritual solution. This approach has streamlined my efforts to assist in healing.

Physical source symptoms can be addressed allopathically, homeopathically, nutritionally, and osteopathically with the judicious use of acupuncture and herbs, both Western and Chinese. The latter fields of understanding and treatment make up the lion's share of the 70 percent. To broaden my abilities, I needed to educate myself on these topics; the only one I have not undertaken is Chinese medicine. A single practitioner cannot master and be proficient in all of these modalities. All learning is ultimately self-learning, and I learned about homeopathy through workshops, a lot of self-study, and specific practitioners I could prevail upon in moments of need.

When patients present with strictly somatic dysfunction, we need to be able to lay hands on their bodies and, with educated fingers, sense the disturbance and correct it. Medical school does not address this work at all. The majority of pain complaints (somatic dysfunction) are treated with narcotics and muscle relaxers, with maybe a referral for physical therapy. We know where this approach often leads, namely narcotic addiction. In trying to help, we often contribute to a huge problem, which is another violation of the Hippocratic Oath. Would it not make more sense to learn a system of healing that involves actually touching the patient with "thinking fingers" and correcting the source of the problem? This is what traditional osteopathy, in particular cranial osteopathy, addresses. The initial training is a weeklong intensive, but to become proficient takes a lifetime. The work deepens with persistent and consistent practice. It takes time, and that is one thing that is almost universally missing today. Other than juggling a patient's medication regimen, little can be accomplished in a five- to ten-minute office visit. A solid osteopathic treatment, from a cranial perspective, takes at least a half-hour; this does not include the time it takes to get a proper history. How many physicians take this kind of time to listen both with their minds and their fingers? Very few.

Between my allopathic, homeopathic, nutritional, and lifestyle understanding, my success rate with patients is at least 80 percent, and I am still getting better. This is a percentage I can live with, but it is no cause for hubris. So much remains that is mysterious and beyond my understanding; staying humble is a prerequisite for what is unknown to become known.

DOWSING

At one of the early AHMA meetings, I attended a presentation on dowsing. I had no idea what a dowser was at the time, but what the lecturer presented was fascinating. Dowsing, or "water witching," has been practiced for centuries. A dowser cuts a willow or hazel branch in the shape of a Y. While holding on to the two "forks" with the single part of the branch parallel to the ground, they walk over the earth. When the dowser passes over underground water, the stick is strongly forced toward the ground. Both the spot and the depth of the water are noted, and sure enough, drilling will confirm the dowser's finding. No one really understands how this works, but we know that it does. Even oil companies employ dowsers to assist in discovery. The talk was so fascinating, I wound up speaking with the presenter and purchasing his book afterward. In the book, there is a chapter on map dowsing. Apparently, some dowsers can find underground water using a pendulum and a topographic map. If it were not for the fact that they can do this, it would seem too far-fetched. That dowsing was capable of accomplishing the same results remotely was even more so.

I was not interested in finding underground water, but I was very interested in discovering a patient's medical information. Could I learn to use a pendulum to access it? Instead of a topographic map, I would write down all of my questions and use the pendulum over what was written. More importantly, I found dowsing to be extremely useful for effectuating my triage. Is the source of a given problem physical, mental/emotional, or spiritual? I discovered that the pendulum could help provide that answer.

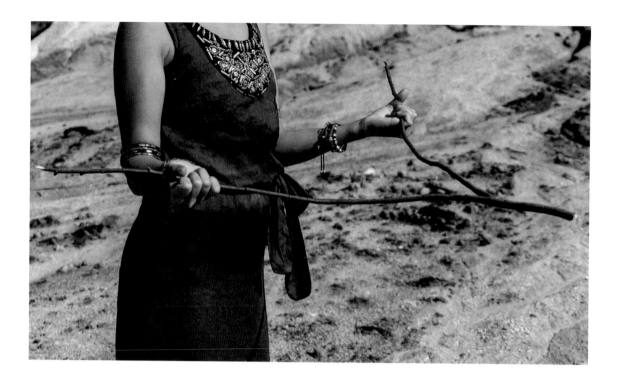

A few words are needed here to help you understand what a pendulum is and what it can help with. First, not all pendulums are functional; in fact, most are not, and if you tried to dowse with one of these, nothing would happen. Most crystal pendulums aspire to look good but are useless for dowsing.

A small (1- to 1½-inch) plumb bob or metal ball with a point on the bottom (about ¾ inch) with about 1 foot of string is perfect for dowsing. These are both sensitive and active with the subtle energies we are trying to detect. Pendulum dowsing is an extremely sensitive feedback mechanism where we are simply looking for movement, usually circular but sometimes back and forth, to affirm our question. It is a binary affair: movement is a "yes," and no movement is a "no."

One must be as neutral as possible when putting forth a question. True neutrality takes many years of practice and can be quite tricky. By the very act of formulating a question, we often have an inkling of an answer (our bias), and the pendulum will affirm that bias. This is of no help. Bias prevents neutrality, and without neutrality, effective dowsing is impossible. Cultivating neutrality and thereby getting proficiency is a lifelong affair. It can be frustrating and slow-going in the beginning; it was for me.

The best way to describe how dowsing works is that all information is already "out there," often in the form of energy waves. Consider all of the radio stations broadcasting 24/7, but we never know about them until we turn on the radio and a whole new world of sound magically appears. The waves of information are out there, but we need a receiver to make this information known. I believe we are all broadcasting the energetic truth of our being 24/7, and using a pendulum can help us "hear" it. I'm sure there are other ways to access this information, but dowsing has worked for me for forty years. It is not for everyone, but for those with a natural affinity and an ability to stay neutral, the pendulum can help gather information that may be hard to get in other ways.

For me, the symptoms were either physical or mental/emotional in origin for many years; spiritual origin never came up, until one day it did. I realized that I was not sure what precisely "spiritual" even meant. Was it related to God or to one's religion? Was it related to a spiritual malady? How could I find out what it meant? I started writing my "map" over which I could dowse. I wrote down everything I could think of, but I got no positive readings. After much time and effort, what I came to was that a spiritual origin of a symptom or disease has nothing to do with God or religious sensibilities. It has to do with the energy matrix of the body, independent of physical or mental/emotional causes—specifically, energy that is not our own, yet is stuck or glommed on to our energy matrix. A common illusion is that we are fully autonomous and independent energy systems. The truth is that we interact energetically with others all the time, but in most cases the outside energy goes home when the party is over. Think of the union of energies that occurs during lovemaking and the mingling of energies that occurs during expressions of empathy and compassion; these unions do not cause problems. It is only when an outside energy gets stuck in our matrix that a problem arises. And it can be a real humdinger. It's like a house guest who refuses to leave and wants to take over your house, or a computer virus that slows your operating system or shuts it down entirely.

I would like to think that these events are not by design or done with the intent to harm, but I know that they can be and has historically been done to harm or even to destroy. In this day and age, most of these situations seem to be related to jealousy. Jealousy is like Velcro to our energy matrix; it is the stickiest of emotions. There are many ways that unwanted energies can get stuck in/on us, but that energy requires some sort of spoken or unspoken permission in order to invade. This process is often unconscious, and I am able to simply approach a person (or map dowse) with my pendulum to detect this "energy virus."

For the vast majority of patients who give their history, the source of their problem is revealed within the first ten to fifteen minutes of their visit. After forty years of listening to patients' stories, I know that most stories are variations on a theme and are readily recognizable. When I hear a story that simply makes no sense, I am alerted to the possibility of an energetic virus as the origin of the problem. Dowsing quickly confirms whether this is true.

When Patient X gave their history, the story did not add up, and the dots just did not connect. After I determined what a spiritual origin to a problem really meant for this patient, I needed to figure out what to do about it. I had no one to consult; I needed to find out for myself. Again, I wrote out my map from which I could dowse. I first had to ascertain that I could actually do something to help the patient resolve their energetic virus. I found that I could indeed. I then wrote out every therapeutic modality I could think of. I got no positive response. I wrote down all of the therapies that I knew about, but I was neither knowledgeable nor proficient with any of them. I got a strong positive reading with my pendulum over "sound therapy." What sound could it be? A sound from nature or possibly from a musical instrument? The pendulum swung wildly over musical instrument. I wrote down every orchestral instrument known to me with no positive result. Then I wrote down every other type of instrument I could think of. When I got to the didgeridoo, my pendulum went wild. I determined that the didgeridoo was to be played over this person's body, creating a vibratory effect. Knowing that these instruments come in a single note, I determined that the D note would be the most effective at removing the unwanted energy.

Learning to play the didgeridoo was my next project. I was thankful that the pendulum did not point to the violin or cello. Learning those at my age would not have been pretty. But I figured I could blow into a hollow stick and make sounds. It was not quite as easy as I had anticipated, but I got the hang of it.

These concepts, when explained to patients, are surprisingly readily understood and accepted. Having a "didge" session feels great and can be profound. It invariably removes the unwanted energy. If a patient comes back repeatedly with the same problem, we need to look at how they are rolling out the red carpet for unwanted energy.

Most are unaware that they are doing so and can change their behavior when it is pointed out.

It is enough to ascertain a spiritual origin to a problem or disease and then to clear the energetic matrix with the didgeridoo. It is usually not necessary to explore exactly how and why the matrix lost its autonomy. Those who are able to dig deep into these matters will most certainly be rewarded for their efforts.

I'd like to share a story from one of my patients, Elaine, about her healing experience with didgeridoo sound therapy. Elaine wrote:

I have had many experiences with the didgeridoo. It helps remove my blocked energy and releases it.

One of my most memorable experiences:

I was walking with my mother over a grassy area in a shopping center. As we walked, an unusual energy shot up from the soles of my feet to the top of my head. It made my hair stand straight up; it was a very uncomfortable feeling. We proceeded to go shopping. When we were leaving, not paying attention, I walked over the same area, and again it happened. By the time I got home about twenty minutes later, I could barely get out of the car.

This energy made me physically sick for a few weeks. I became unable to walk without excruciating pain in my legs and back. In my first appointment with Dr. D, we talked in depth while he took notes. With his dowsing, he was able to tell me what had transpired and what I had picked up while on that grassy area. The energy was not my own. The dowsing gave us information on how to remove the energy, but the didgeridoo was the sacred instrument used to help remove this heavy energy, and I felt much better immediately.

Oftentimes when my own energy is low, I seem to pick up unwanted energy. If I let this unwanted energy hang around, I can't sleep and I am so agitated, and others around me feel that something is off. Dr. D will recheck with the dowser and determine if [the energy] is from a spiritual source. Then I lie on the table, and he checks which note of the didgeridoo will be used to remove the unwanted energy. Within a few minutes, it's gone, and I feel like myself again.

I have another patient, Jennifer, who has allowed me to share her remarkable and transformative story that incorporates dowsing and the use of the didgeridoo and a deep act of forgiveness and redemption:

Jenn showed up at my office looking sad and concerned. "How can I help?" I asked. She said she needed some Valium, just enough to get her through the holidays. I asked her to expound on this, and she told me that every year since 1987, she became suicidal and depressed at Christmastime; after the New Year, she snapped out of it and was perfectly fine until the next Christmas. Many people feel sad during the holidays, but becoming suicidal for a couple of weeks is very disturbing. I asked her what happened in 1987. Casually, she said that on Christmas Eve, a man had raped her in her home…under her own Christmas tree, which she was just finishing decorating. She recognized him as a jogger in the neighborhood.

"I knew my husband and son were on their way home, and all I could think was, I hope he gets through with this quickly so my son does not have to deal with this. When he was done, he went to the kitchen. I thought he might try to kill me with my own kitchen knife, and he would have the fight of his life if he tried. But he came back with some damp cloths and gently cleaned me up. I was very confused by this. As he left, I ran to get my .45 and went after him. As I drew a bead on his back, I realized the gun was unloaded. With a child in the house, I was careful to hide the ammunition. I would have shot the rapist if the gun had been loaded, but I was not meant to kill him. He took care of that himself, dying by suicide three weeks later. I thought at the time that it was all over, but year after year at Christmas, when I see the decorations going up, these feelings of sadness, deep despair, fear, confusion, and suicidal thoughts arise. Every year, I take Valium,

and it eases me along until the New Year arrives."

At this point, I did my dowsing and got a spiritual origin for her depression. I asked if I could help her in a deeper way than prescribing a tranquilizer. I explained that I could sweep her body with the didge, and we'd see what happened. Jenn described her didge session as "almost like a massage from the inside out, vibrating things so they can be released." She loved the experience and went home without Valium. We did not have to wait long to see what would happen next.

The next morning, Jenn was agitated and knew she needed to go back to the doctor. When she arrived at my office, she grabbed me and would not let go; she was in a state. "You have to help me!" she pleaded. I asked her husband to go up to the office and bring my assistant Jody down to us. I sensed in Jenn a rising energy about to erupt, and I needed reinforcements. Jody was needed to ground the experience, and when Jenn saw her, she let me go and clung to Jody instead. Jenn did not let her go for the next hour.

We laid Jenn down on my treatment table. She was full-body sobbing and reported an odd feeling in her abdomen that she had never felt before. Being held tightly and being very much the empath, Jody could feel this odd sensation as well. I began quietly coaching Jody to ask key questions. When Jody asked Jenn what was wrong, Jenn said this guy would not stop bothering her. "He raped me, then killed himself. I thought that it was all over. But it's not. I felt compelled to hold on to Jody, thinking that if she let go of me, I was going to go somewhere and never come back." Jenn's husband was petrified that this might happen.

No one knew what was about to transpire, but we all knew it was something big, and at least two of us were concerned about Jenn's return. I wasn't, but I knew we needed to see this to its completion no matter how long it took.

Jenn described the experience this way: "Jody grounded me, and at that moment, an intense energy erupted from me, and I left my body. I was flying through space so fast with not a hint of resistance. I did not even know you could go that fast. Stars were going by me; it seemed like I was traveling at lightspeed like in *Star Wars*. Then, kerplunk—I was in complete darkness. This place was so dark, so sad, with total hopelessness and despair. You would not wish this place on your worst enemy. I slowly realized there was another spirit with me; I did not 'see' it with my eyes, but rather sensed it with my whole being. I knew it was the rapist, and he was in terrible despair. I told him that he could not stay there and that we needed to leave. No one else was there…just the two of us in a place of no light and no love. I turned to my right, and there was what appeared to be a beautiful full moon; the light was overpowering. When I faced away from the light, all I could sense was complete darkness; it was as if there was complete darkness next to complete light, but the light did not penetrate the darkness, nor did the darkness penetrate the light. I learned in that moment that there is no darkness without light and no light without darkness. I always have a choice to either face the darkness or face the light. We can always choose.

"[The rapist] felt so bad about himself, and I realized that while he was responsible for all the pain inflicted on me and others, he himself was horribly tormented and damaged. I could sense that he was not a bad person. I begged him to let me help him to the light. He said he could not. It was strange that I felt only love for him in spite of what he had done to me. Here we were in this darkness; I was aware of this light, and I was begging him to come with me into that light. He was so out of place, yet he belonged there in the dark. He did not want to go to the light; he felt he did not deserve to go. 'Listen to me. I love you, and I forgive you. You need to move to the light,' I told him. He said that he was not worthy, that he had no business going into the light. We went back and forth with no result.

"At this point, I was lying on the table with Jody leaning over my head, her hand on my belly. I noticed that her neck was pulsating. I reached for the amulet around her neck and sensed that I needed to hold this gift from her grandmother who was a lay healer. Immediately, I saw the wispiest angel fabric moving wavelike from the light into the darkness where we were. It came and encircled us. I begged for her (I knew it was Jody's grandmother) to help move him to the light. Together, we tried, but he was so scared and felt so horrible about himself. I heard Jody's grandmother say that we needed more help. She traveled back to the light and shortly returned with many more wispy things that I assumed were angels. They encircled us and started to move us toward the light. He continued to resist, but I told him that we loved him and if you have love, you do not belong in the darkness. So much energy and so much love. A big white ring surrounded us, and he went right into the light; it was over."

"I was back in my body on the table and completely exhausted; it was an exhaustion I had never known. It was like I was reborn, and I was a little baby. I had to be carried to the car and brought home. I was free of anxiety and fear. The grand finale was a hot Hawaiian salt bath. This experience marked the end of my annual suicidal depression. I can celebrate and have fun and not have an ounce of sadness." Jenn has had about fifteen years of freedom from her winter anguish.

Jenn had some reflections that she wanted to share: "If there is forgiveness and self-forgiveness, everyone ends up in the light. Everyone. But not everyone wants to be. The light always wants us to come back in, but it is our choice. I could not heal until I forgave [my attacker] and helped him to the light. It was up to me the whole time. Who knew?"

There is so much richness to comment on, but I will only touch on the catalyst of this spontaneous experience. Dowsing pointed me in the right direction. Jenn did not need medication or psychotherapy; she had tried a lot of both with no effect. Her issue was spiritual, and the pendulum led us to didgeridoo sound therapy. I actually blew four different didges (notes) over her body. I started with D, which cleanses and activates the solar plexus, and then used E, which has its action over the heart region. Then I used F, which affects the neck, and finished with G, which affects the head and made her laugh. The net effect was to clear energetic blockages and catalyze the experience that followed.

There are other ways to get to that point (Reichian Breathwork, Bioenergetics, and Holotropic Breathwork, to name a few), but in this extraordinary example, dowsing and the didgeridoo combined to energize a life-changing experience for Jenn. It has remained the peak experience of her life.

POSSESSION AND THE EXISTENCE OF EVIL FORCES

Separate from Jenn's experience, I have had several other interactions with patients in which their illness appeared to stem from what we might call "possession." These events opened up an ongoing exploration of good and evil in my work. It soon became apparent that there is what I call both endogenous and exogenous evil—meaning there is evil within us and evil that comes from outside of us.

Solzhenitsyn stated clearly in *The Gulag Archipelago* that the line between good and evil runs through every human heart. It is only through ongoing vigilance and choice that we can expand the light and shrink the darkness. We can also go the other way: expanding the darkness and shrinking the light. This speaks to the endogenous form of evil, and we all can relate to this internal struggle. There seem to be two opposing voices in our heads: a voice of light and a voice of darkness. Which voice we listen to determines our fate.

The existence of an evil force or entity outside of ourselves is hard to fathom and, as such, can fill us with fear and dread. We think such thoughts as, "Am I doing my best to live a good life?" "Under what circumstances can this lurking danger grab me?" And "what, if anything, can I do to prevent this or deal with it if it intrudes on my life?" Meaty questions indeed. Humans always seem to have lived with the uncertainty of an outside force ending their lives. Whether in the form of a marauding tribe, illness, or climate catastrophe, external forces have always been there and probably always will be.

We have developed many skills to cope with uncertainty from the physical realm: medicines and surgery to ward off and treat illness, strong communities to withstand outside attacks, and technologies that shelter us from the whims of nature. But a force of evil from the outside presents an unseen spiritual challenge. Few of us seem to know how to understand and contextualize it, or how to deal with it when we are affected. It also begs the question of just how commonly it occurs. How many among us are walking around with a compromised energy matrix (possession)? What are the consequences?

My experience informs me that possession is far more common than I ever thought. It is far from a rare occurrence. Fortunately, however, it is usually easily and quickly remedied when identified.

While this entire subject may seem bizarre, it must be recognized that possession has been an ongoing subject of discussion from the beginning of recorded history. The manner of discussion and the various treatments attempted have varied, but it has always had a place at the spiritual table. In our modern age, this discussion may seem archaic, but it is as relevant now as it was in any preceding period. There is a need to inquire and identify it as an operative theme in a patient's life. Then, once we know it is there, we can clear it away and clean the energy matrix with sound healing. Where does this energy go when removed from the body? Back to wherever it came from. The mysteries of spirit run deep, and awe seems to be the appropriate response to the grandeur and mystery of our life.

To further expand this discussion, I would like to describe a formative experience from my first year of medical practice. After completing my internship and work in the Indian Health Service, I was asked to care for a young woman who complained of severe and uncontrollable seizures. Her husband accompanied her to my clinic, and both explained that she had seen many neurologists and had tried many medications and forms of treatment from university medical centers but continued to experience severe, daily seizures that left her exhausted and unable to function. These seizures were so bizarre that the couple had on two occasions asked a Catholic priest who was skilled in this area to attempt exorcisms for what they felt was possession. The exorcisms had not worked.

Other than what I had read in books and seen in movies, I had no knowledge of possession. I am Jewish, so it was not a part of my religious education, either. Honestly, I was skeptical…I thought it to be a somewhat convenient explanation for her condition, but trying all of my skills (which, admittedly, were limited in those days), I was not of much help. They came to trust me, so one day, they asked me to be present, as their medical representative, at another attempt at exorcism by a Catholic priest. While it was completely outside of my comfort zone, I was intrigued at the opportunity to witness this ceremony, and hoped I could be of some help if needed (although what kind of help I could give, I did not know).

The ritual was to be performed in my office, in the evening. The principals assembled, and soon after the priest began chanting, in Latin, some form of invocation, my patient began writhing in a way similar to several seizures I had witnessed in my office, but then she began grunting, screaming, and making ear-splitting and unearthly noises. Within a few minutes, a dark presence manifested in the room: an overwhelming sense of power and doom. It was like nothing I had ever experienced, and I had no idea what to do; I was terrified. I had no training, skills, or knowledge of how to process this experience. Filled with fear, I crawled under a table in the corner, assumed the fetal position, and prayed, covering myself with what I imagined to be white light. The chanting and screaming went on for seemed like hours (but probably lasted about forty-five minutes), during which time my only focus was on my own safety. Finally, the ordeal abated. My patient was dripping with sweat, pale, and exhausted. So was the priest. I was just glad it was over. I had never felt so useless.

I followed this patient medically for several months afterward. The attempt at exorcism was unsuccessful, and her seizures continued. Eventually, she left the area and was lost to my medical care.

I present this story to you as a cautionary tale. I am, and have always been, an optimistic person. In my naivete, I assumed that with good intentions and a belief in God, and with my medical knowledge, I could be of help. I was not. Hundreds of books are filled with visualizations and affirmations of how the power of love and light, filled with good intentions, can change anything for the good and for healing.

Be careful. This experience woke me up to how little I knew of the forces of good and/or evil and about energies. We should enter into areas of this nature only under the guidance of those with the proper training, experience, and knowledge.

This is a beautiful example of how "fools rush in where angels fear to tread." Been there, done that. If you are going to work with energies, be sure they are benign.

Please understand that in this world, there is evil. There are malevolent forces. Some people try to spiritually brush this aside as a manifestation of the jealousy and rage of those who feel they have been wronged or slighted. While understanding this may be a kind and compassionate approach, it can also lull you into not appreciating the depth of the energetic damage it can do to you if you are blindsided. Enter into these realms with your eyes wide open and with humility, and stay protected.

Because of the charged topic of "possession," Dr. D wishes to remain anonymous.

CHAPTER 12:

Acupuncture and the Perception of Qi

Let's Get to the Point

Acupuncture is one is the oldest healing traditions. *The Yellow Emperor's Classic of Internal Medicine* was written in about 2600 BC and for centuries served as a model for diagnosis and treatment in China. I mentioned my own experience with acupuncture earlier in this book (see page 75). I would add that in addition to studying with a Chinese acupuncturist who worked in our office one day a week, I studied with Efrem Korngold, LAc, and Felix Mann, MD, two of the practitioners who helped bring this discipline to the West.

Many Westerners associate acupuncture exclusively with the placement of needles over acupuncture points on the body, but the practice is far more extensive than needling. A prescription from a practitioner of traditional Chinese medicine is just as likely to include exercises (tai chi and qi gong), meditation, and an extensive herbal pharmaceutical compendium.

Central to this discipline is the palpation and perception of energy flows in a person who comes for treatment. The word for energy in Chinese is *chi* or *qi;* in Japanese it is *ki.* Feeling the energy flows, or blockages to those flows, is primarily done by taking a "pulse." While this effort is superficially similar to how a medical doctor takes a pulse by placing a finger alongside the wrist, the similarity ends there. Physicians are taught simply to feel for the number of heartbeats per minute and assess force and regularity. In practice, however, the pulse at a conventional physician's office is taken by a nurse, if at all, and only the rate is noted. Physicians rarely take the pulse themselves, thereby missing out on a great deal of information.

Acupuncture takes the act of feeling the pulse to much higher levels. Three fingers are placed over the radial artery on each wrist, and each finger feels a different quality of pulse, first gently and then more deeply. With this setup, each finger is able to register the energy flowing through the six different acupuncture meridians (channels of energy flow) on each wrist, which provides information on the twelve basic meridian flow patterns. That is just the beginning. Advanced practitioners can feel up to forty different qualities of pulse, which allows them to make a detailed diagnosis of energy flow in a patient and know how to stimulate or quiet those flows when they are out of balance.

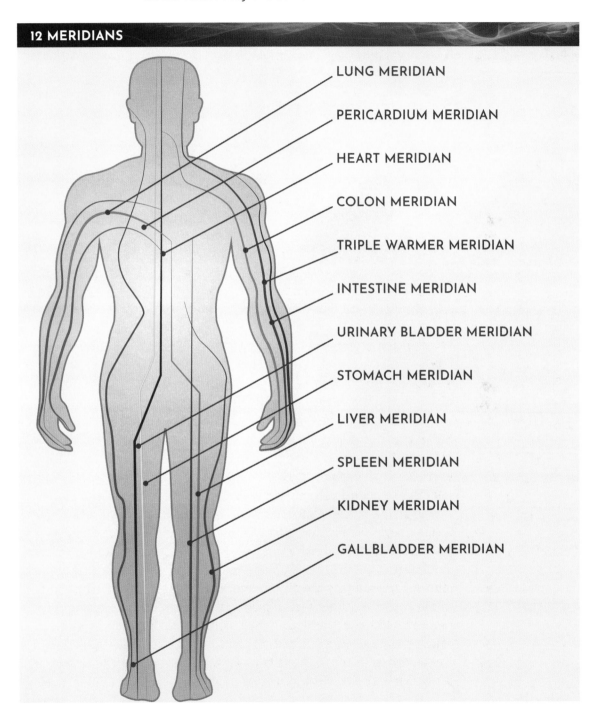

12 MERIDIANS

LUNG MERIDIAN

PERICARDIUM MERIDIAN

HEART MERIDIAN

COLON MERIDIAN

TRIPLE WARMER MERIDIAN

INTESTINE MERIDIAN

URINARY BLADDER MERIDIAN

STOMACH MERIDIAN

LIVER MERIDIAN

SPLEEN MERIDIAN

KIDNEY MERIDIAN

GALLBLADDER MERIDIAN

A second area of study in Chinese medicine is a patient's tongue. While conventional medicine does teach this process, it is not as elaborate as the Chinese process, in which many aspects of tongue physiology provide information about a patient's health and vitality.

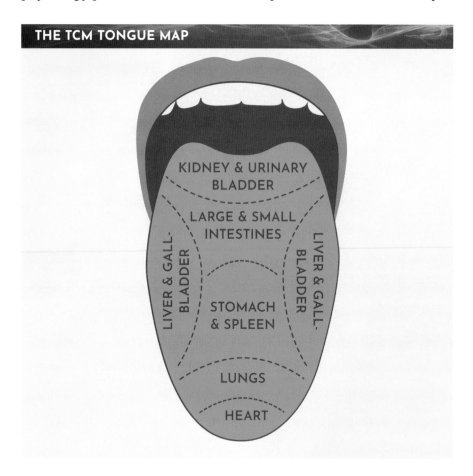

THE TCM TONGUE MAP

KIDNEY & URINARY BLADDER

LARGE & SMALL INTESTINES

LIVER & GALL-BLADDER

LIVER & GALL-BLADDER

STOMACH & SPLEEN

LUNGS

HEART

Although acupuncture was an early mainstay of my practice, as more and more acupuncturists were trained in Chinese medicine, I began to refer more and more patients to my colleagues. To be completely honest, my acupuncture, while often effective, was rather "cookbook" in its practice. What I mean is that I used well-established patterns of placement for acupuncture needles to treat pain rather than relying on (or getting good at) feeling the energies required to do this practice optimally. Therefore, I felt I should turn over the writing of this chapter to someone with more current and in-depth hands-on practice.

I have had the pleasure of working with Emily Rowe, MD, for several years now and have found her knowledge of Traditional Chinese Medicine and its use in healing to be exceptional. She begins by showing us how even the Chinese characters for qi reflect the inherent perception of energy, and then blends this into how we can integrate this information with a knowledge of the science underlying these observations. Her detailed description of what acupuncture is, from an energy perspective, follows.

WHAT IS QI?

by EMILY ROWE, MD

Qi is a Chinese medical concept that I find difficult to articulate in English. It is pronounced "chee," as in the first part of the word *cheese.* I find it helpful to look at the Chinese character to understand what is meant by the term *qi.*

The Modern Chinese character for qi is 氣. It consists of two parts. The bottom portion is "mi" 米, which means rice. The word for rice looks like an asterisk with eight directions, which is a reference to the Ba Gua 八卦, the Eight Trigrams or Eight Directions. The Ba Gua are the eight symbols used in Taoist cosmology to represent the fundamental principles of reality, the physical world. The character mi 米 represents an idea of nourishment, which is centering (the middle of the eight directions) and grounds us in reality. The top portion of the character is yun 云, which is a simplification of the word for cloud. So the character for qi is literally the image of clouds of steam coming off of rice.

The character for qi 氣 evokes an image. Personally, I see a process of sublimation, which is a chemistry term that describes moving from a solid state directly to a gaseous state, skipping the liquid phase. This process occurs based on the environmental temperature and pressure. When heat is applied to a solid material, its molecules absorb the heat and start to vibrate more quickly. The excited molecules can vibrate so quickly that they start to move away from one another, and they are sublimed into the atmosphere. So the character for qi is about taking nourishment from the eight directions and sublimating it—taking the material and making it immaterial. So the character qi 氣 indicates a process of changing states.

The word *qi* does not mean energy! This is a mistranslation. *Qi is about the relationship between the material and the immaterial, the process of changing from grounded tangible reality into something sublime.*

HOW DOES ONE PERCEIVE QI?

According to Chinese medicine, qi runs through meridians, or channels in the body. Take a look at an acupuncture model, with lines running over the surface of the body. The lines run vertically along the arms and legs, zigzagging and crisscrossing at various points, creating a web of "roads" along which qi can travel.

The modern-day analogy is that acupuncture meridians are qi highways in the body, but the acupuncture model doesn't show everything. It shows only the surface of the body. Chinese medical textbooks demonstrate the internal dives that each acupuncture meridian makes toward the internal organs. As an acupuncture student, I spent long hours memorizing the channels and points, the connections between the meridians and the body locations where multiple meridians cross. The qi highway metaphor is useful as an explanation for how acupuncture works. How can a point on your leg affect your organs of digestion? Well, the point on the leg travels to and connects to the stomach and intestines. So when this point is massaged, you can hear your intestines start to rumble. My husband and I used to laugh in Chinese medical school because every time I pressed on his Large Intestine point LI-10 on his forearm, he would fart.

This highway metaphor was useful when I was a student studying the anatomy of qi in books. But once I started needling, I began to understand another image used in ancient China. The meridians were thought of as waterways, not highways, for the travel of qi within the body. Ancient China didn't have a highly developed highway system, but it had a sophisticated canal system, and goods were run through the canals and along the Yangtze and Huai rivers. The Chinese medical image of qi flowing through the acupuncture channels is that of water bubbling up from a spring and becoming a stream, which leads to a river and finally pours out into the sea.

Imagine that as you manipulate points with acupuncture, you are guiding a boat down these waterways, allowing it smooth passage. So, with an acupuncture treatment, you help to "course the waterways." Metaphorically, you might remove a rock that is blocking a spring from bubbling up out of the ground. Removing the rock restores the flow of water downstream. Or you might move a log out of the way of a river so that a boat can get easily get by. In some cases, there might be a dam over an acupuncture channel. And when you look at a channel, you don't just assess the water; you also assess the surrounding terrain. Are the banks of the river a soggy mess, with stagnant water like a marsh?

This flow of qi is perceived in a variety of ways. As I run my fingers over an acupuncture channel, I ask myself, "What is the terrain of this acupuncture channel?" It is almost like assessing the terroir for a particular wine. Terroir is a concept in wine tasting where the climate, weather, and environment of the land on which the grapes are grown impart a unique flavor to the wine. It can change from year to year, depending on the amount of rain or sun the area gets or the mineral content of the soil. Similarly, when you assess an acupuncture meridian, you are looking at the terroir of the qi.

COLLAGEN AND THE PIEZOELECTRIC EFFECT

When I was in Western medical school, I had the privilege of dissecting a cadaver. Donating one's human body so that physicians can learn about the muscles, internal organs, blood vessels, and so on is a great anatomical gift and an irreplaceable educational experience. Each week, we would dissect a different body part and memorize the various structures and connections. Four medical students shared one cadaver. At the end of the dissection, we would walk around the rooms of the gross anatomy lab and look at the anatomical variations among different cadavers. But there was no discussion of collagen, fascia, and connective tissue in my gross anatomy class. Collagen was viewed as "filler," something that was in the way of the actual organs. We cut it away and disregarded it. Our instructors would say, "Get this fascia out of here so that we can see the structure," as we dissected the cadaver.

Fascia was also heedlessly cut and moved out of the way while I observed surgeries two years later. Surgeons cut through the fascia to get to problem areas that lay deeper within the organs. My only recollection of studying the structure of collagen in conventional medical school was during a one-day biochemistry lecture in my first year. It was never discussed again. But collagen is what holds us together! And I believe that collagen is where the qi flows. Collagen constructs the springs, streams, rivers, and seas of the acupuncture meridians.

The chemical structure of collagen consists of three strands of amino acids wound into a triple-helix structure. It is rich in three amino acids: proline, hydroxyproline, and glycine, which form a stable, rigid structure that is just like a crystal's. These triple helical strands of collagen are locked together by hydrogen bonds to form collagen fibers. These are what hold us together and provide us with the gift of structural integrity!

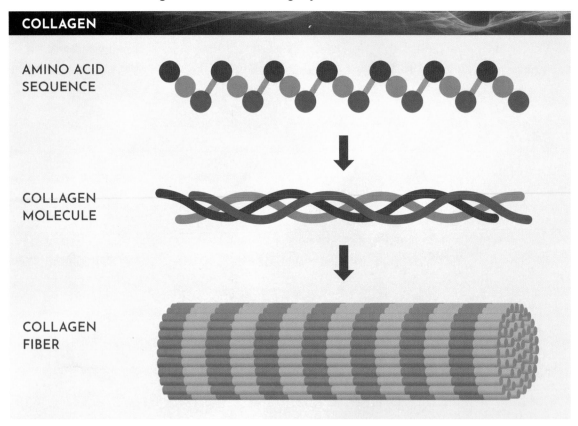

COLLAGEN

AMINO ACID SEQUENCE

COLLAGEN MOLECULE

COLLAGEN FIBER

There are multiple types of collagen in the body. Collagen forms skin, fascia, tendons, bones, cartilage, hair, and placenta. It varies in hardness depending on the level of mineralization. Collagen has enormous tensile strength and is used to form a variety of structures and networks within the body. It is a special protein because it has a property called piezoelectricity: when you press on it, there is an induction of an electric charge. Mechanical stress placed on collagen leads to electricity. And wherever you have electricity, you generate a magnetic field. Within your body, collagen forms a matrix of crystals that can conduct electromagnetic fields while holding you together, generating a network of electromagnetic fields.

Appearance of an electric potential across certain faces of a crystal when it is subjected to mechanical pressure.

Conversely, when an electric field is applied to one of the faces of the crystal it undergoes mechanical distortion.

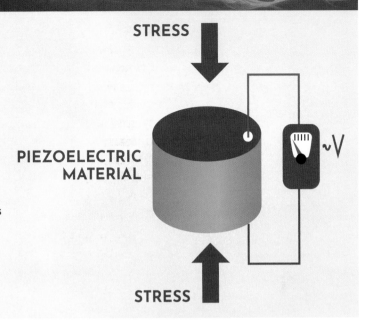

STRESS

PIEZOELECTRIC MATERIAL

~V

STRESS

Some of the first studies of the piezoelectric effect were done in the 1880s by brothers Jacques and Pierre Curie. They studied crystals, such as tourmaline and quartz. Interestingly, they found that quartz exhibited the most piezoelectricity. It wasn't until years later that the piezoelectric effect was understood as part of a biological system. In the 1960s, scientific experiments demonstrated that collagen has a piezoelectric effect. One study found that when a tendon from the leg of an ox was mechanically manipulated, the electrical signal was able to be transmitted to a gramophone. Tendons, which are made of collagen, can act as electromechanical transducers, carrying electrical signals and generating electromagnetic fields.

In Chinese medicine, all of the parts of the body that have piezoelectrical properties, including bones, DNA, collagen, fascia, hair, placenta, and connective tissue, correspond to the deepest jing 精 level. Jing is the medical term for essence. In Chinese medicine, jing evokes the idea of the densest physical matter.

If collagen within our bodies has a crystalline structure, which allows the creation and transduction of electrical signals, then this piezoelectric effect evokes the ancient idea of qi 氣. You are taking a solid object (collagen) and applying mechanical force, which leads to a flow of electrons (electricity). This is a process of taking something material and transforming it into something intangible (the flow of electricity), which is the definition of qi! So, when you press and pull and apply mechanical force to the collagen in the body, a mechanochemical transformation occurs whereby electrical signals can be transduced. And where does this electricity flow? Within networks of collagen! Whenever you have electricity, you generate magnetic fields. Since the electricity cannot be separated from the magnetic field, we call it an electromagnetic field. So your collagen, bones, DNA, fascia, and connective tissues are conduits for electromagnetic fields.

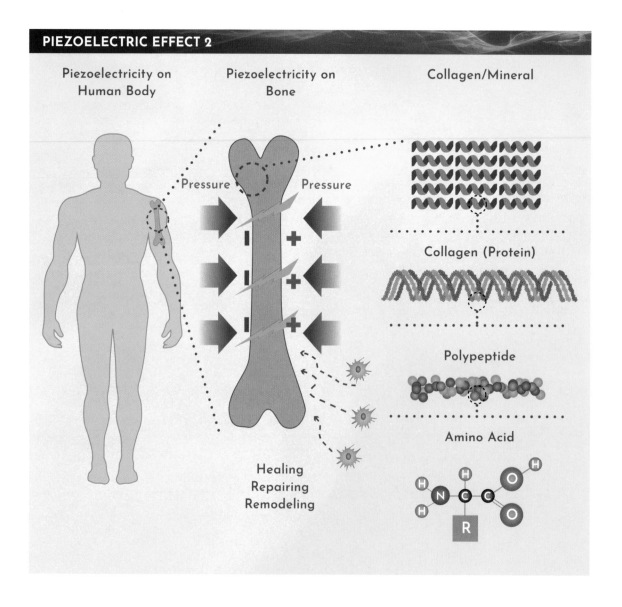

PIEZOELECTRIC EFFECT 2

Piezoelectricity on Human Body

Piezoelectricity on Bone

Collagen/Mineral

Pressure   Pressure

Collagen (Protein)

Polypeptide

Amino Acid

Healing
Repairing
Remodeling

A further interesting aspect of all this is the reverse piezoelectric effect, which means that applying an external electromagnetic field generates internal mechanical strain. So there is a cyclical relationship. This makes me wonder about how all of these electromagnetic fields to which we are currently exposed might be affecting our collagen structures.

What does this mean for my practice? It is my belief that the acupuncture meridians flow within collagen networks. These networks are conduits for electromagnetic fields. So acupuncture, which is the act of applying mechanical force with needles to collagen structures in the body, can stimulate that piezoelectrical scaffolding network to create electrical stimulation and a possible tissue regeneration response! The tissue regeneration response happens as the electromagnetic fields cause physical mechanical changes, triggering the body's innate intelligence to heal. This mechanism of action also explains how qi gong and other martial arts forms can use structure (martial arts stances) to generate qi (electromagnetic fields) by placing stress on the collagen of the body in particular ways.

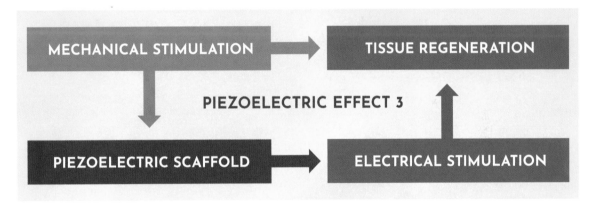

Qi represents that process of moving from a solid state to an intangible state, which is described by the piezoelectric effect. And yet that intangible state can still be sensed! But how do we sense that qi? Let's go back to the image of a cloud coming off of a grain of rice.

A cloud can be perceived and seen, but it is not solid or tangible. Have you ever walked through a mist on a foggy day and felt the heaviness of the air? Have you ever been to a cloud forest where persistent condensation combined with cooling air currents leads to the creation and upward deflection of clouds? Walking through this mist, you can feel the changing chemical states in the air! Or imagine the changes you feel in the air just before a thunderstorm hits. The pressure drops. You can smell the ozone from the thunder and lightning coming in. Somehow, even with your eyes closed, you know that a storm is approaching. Your body senses this weather change— but how? We can all do it, but it's hard to articulate how we know that a storm is rolling in. There is a feeling of heaviness in the atmosphere. The air feels thicker and denser on the skin. Somehow, the receptors on our skin can sense the heaviness of all of the water in the air. We feel a change in pressure in our sinus cavities and the internal hollows of our bones. Our ears might pop from the pressure drop. And all this happens before we actually see the sky darkening.

Often, predicting and sensing weather patterns requires an intimate knowledge of the local environment. For example, I have lived in South Florida for the majority of my life. I can look at the sky, feel the pressure and temperature in the air, and know how the patterns of afternoon storms are going to fall. But when I visited Iceland, I couldn't get a gauge of the weather. Iceland has extreme weather that can change rapidly. I was traveling in rural areas, so I couldn't use my phone to type in the name of a city and get the percent chance of rain for the day. While planning a horseback riding excursion, I asked my Swiss guide if it was going to rain. She looked at the sky. Then she sighed and told me that she didn't understand the patterns of the Icelandic weather, either. She had lived in Iceland for only one year and was still unable to gauge the weather by looking at the sky. She said that the weather apps were useless in rural Iceland, as I had already figured out, and she recommended that I ask a Native Icelander, particularly an older one, who could look at the sky and predict the weather for the day. An intimate understanding of the environment, often acquired through time and exposure, allows us to sense these weather changes. And some individuals seem to be more attuned to this than others, but it is something we can all learn to do.

For me, sensing qi is a similar process to sensing shifts in the weather. It is something we can all do. It is not an esoteric skill; anyone can become versed in it by honing and polishing their intuition. But it takes practice.

When practicing acupuncture, you are feeling, sensing, and manipulating the terrain and terroir of the electromagnetic fields of the body. Wow! Let's stop and think about what an honor and a privilege this is! A special intimacy is created when someone asks you to manipulate their qi and shift their electromagnetic fields, and a deep trust must be shared. I am perpetually amazed by the body's innate ability to heal itself when given a push in the right direction. Removing blockages in the collagen, restoring the flow of the electromagnetic fields, and circulating the qi can have enormous health benefits. Once those acupuncture channels are open and the waterways are coursing properly, pain is relieved, anxiety is reduced, and homeostasis begins to return.

This opens up so many questions. There are hundreds of acupuncture points, so how do you go about deciding which points to use? And once you have decided on the points, how do you manipulate them? Do you use needles, or do you change the structure of the body with dietary therapy? Do you use crystals to shift the external electromagnetic fields to induce a reverse piezoelectric process? Do you effect the organs internally through the use of herbs?

Let's go back to that image of waterways. Is a large stone blocking a spring from coming out of the ground? Or maybe there isn't enough water, and what should be a gushing spring is only a tiny trickle. Or maybe the stream is filled with toxins dumped farther upstream from an organ. How do you make a diagnosis and decide what to do?

DIAGNOSING PROBLEMS WITH QI IN CHINESE MEDICINE

In Chinese medical school, students are taught the "four methods of diagnosis," si zhen 四診. Si 四 is the character for the number four, and zhen 診 means to examine a patient. The Chinese character for zhen is interesting. On the left is yan 言, the character for speech (you can see a mouth with vibrations expanding out, making the sounds of speech); on the right is the character for ren 人, a person, with the hair hanging down, shan 彡. This image makes me think of having a talk with a shaman with her hair hanging long.

The root of Chinese medicine is shamanistic. The Chinese character for a shaman is wu 巫. This character has a horizontal line above it, which is heaven, and a horizontal line below it, which is Earth, with a vertical line connecting the two. And then you have the symbol for ren 人, a person, repeated twice. So the character for shaman illustrates someone who is able to be both in heaven and on Earth, connecting the two realms. A shaman has the ability to be in multiple planes of reality. It is about being a conduit, bringing information down from heaven and back to Earth. Taoist shamans traditionally were women who were pictured with their hair hanging down. This image of hair 彡 in the Chinese character for examining a patient, zhen 診, creates a metaphor for the sixth sense involved in this process of examination and diagnosis.

There is a belief in many Native cultures that hair is a physical extension of one's thoughts and allows for extrasensory perception of the environment. Native American trackers were recruited into the US military from World War II until the Vietnam War era for their superior abilities in tracking, which could be useful in combating guerrilla warfare. But once they joined, they were required to have their hair shorn. After their hair was cut, they claimed that their ability to track was diminished because they'd been severed from the precognitive powers that their long hair provided.

The Chinese describe the nature of being human as being caught between heaven and earth. And the three major energies of the body in Chinese medicine reflect this: jing 精, qi 氣, and shen 神. Jing essence is your DNA, your ancestry, your bones—what grounds you in reality and gives you physical form. Shen reflects the intangible things inside you: lightness, spirit, and more. Shen reflects the embodiment of your consciousness, thoughts, and emotions. It is within each of us. For me, the hair, which is a reflection of the shen, is a type of antenna for extrasensory perception. And remember that hair is made of collagen. It can conduct that reverse piezoelectric effect, bringing electromagnetic information from the environment straight into the scalp in the form of mechanical changes! This extrasensory perception, which is represented by long hair, is crucial when examining a patient and coming up with a diagnosis.

Going back to the si zhen 四診, the "four methods of diagnosis," these include

- Observation

- Auscultation and olfaction (this is the same word with a dual meaning in Chinese)

- Interrogation

- Pulse feeling and palpation

Let's look at these techniques and the process that happens in each one.

OBSERVATION

When I first observe a client coming into my clinic, I try to evaluate them based upon wu xing 五, which is Chinese five-element or five-phase theory. This theory was developed in China during the time of the Warring states when philosophers were observing the natural world. The five elements in Chinese medicine are wood, fire, earth, metal, and water. Some people argue that "phase" is a better translation, as the word *xing* 行 indicates a process of moving, traveling, and circulating, not a physical substance, but most English references use "element." Each of us possesses all five elements, and ideally they are in balance.

Picture a carousel with five horses spinning. For the carousel to spin smoothly, all five horses need to be in balance. If one horse is a huge, heavy Clydesdale and another is a miniature pony, the carousel is going to wobble with each spin. To have health and a smooth spin of your carousel in life, you need a balance of all five elements. One element should not be dominant over the others. But most people coming into my clinic have an imbalance; otherwise, they wouldn't need Chinese medicine.

In five-element theory, one element can become another. We call this the generation cycle. When you burn wood, it turns into ashes (earth). You can dig in the earth to find metal. When metal is heated and cooled, water condenses on the outside of it. Metal instruments were also used in ancient cultures to dowse for water located within the earth. And when you water plants and seedlings, they grow, and you get wood! So each element can generate the next one; it a progression from one phase to another.

There is also a control cycle in which one element can balance another. For example, a metal saw can cut down a tree. Water can put out a fire. Wood can break up the soil (earth) and deplete its nutrients. Fire can melt metal. And earth can create a dam to control the flow of water. So ideally, there is a balance between the generation and control cycles.

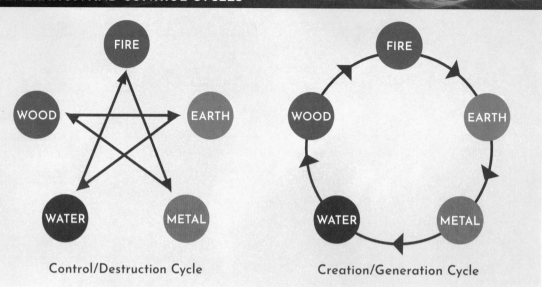

Control/Destruction Cycle   Creation/Generation Cycle

When someone comes into my clinic, I use observation skills to determine which element might be dominant or deficient. Hearing how a person phrases a complaint can give you a big clue as to which element(s) are unbalanced. Often, multiple elements are affected.

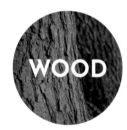

WOOD

Wood is associated with the East direction, spring, growth, regeneration, and the color green. The traditional animal for wood in Chinese culture is the Green Dragon. The East is the direction of the rising sun, representing a new beginning. Wood wants to grow upward toward heaven. Think of spring when the leaves start to sprout out of the barren winter soil. Sprouts have a strong wood energy, springing out of the confined seed, climbing up toward the sunshine. Symbolic of that upward momentum, wood people love goals and feel a sense of accomplishment when they attain a target. They have high aspirations. When a person has evolved their wood element to a high level, they can elevate to high places and look down below. They gain perspective.

The image I like best for "evolved wood" is that of the Condor animal spirit, which represents the direction of the East in Native South American cultures. Imagine this scenario. You are on the way to the airport to catch a flight and you get stuck in a terrible traffic jam. Some idiot driver has blocked traffic for miles! Your irritation and frustration mount as you sit there unmoving, knowing that you are going to miss your flight. The pressure builds. You might even develop elevated blood pressure. Finally, the traffic breaks, you get through the gridlock, you make it to the airport, and you've missed your flight! Luckily, the airline has put you on the next flight, and you have to wait only briefly. You get bumped into first class (wood people love first class!). As you take off and look out the window, you can see the houses, highways, and cars below, and it seems so peaceful. You are above it all. You have perspective on how tiny and unimportant everything seems. You no longer feel the frustration of the traffic. You can see that the "idiot driver" who blocked the traffic had no option to move their car. The turf on the side of the road has collapsed into a ditch next to the road.

That sense of frustration and exasperation, being unable to move toward the place you want to be, is associated with wood imbalances. "Evolved wood" is that higher perspective of the Condor—looking down at the traffic jam from above and having true perspective allows the evolution of compassion. You can truly see what is happening to others, and you have compassion. Unevolved or developing wood personalities are easily irritated and frequently struggle with chronic frustration. I often diagnose wood disharmonies based on someone's level of irritability and frustration. Whereas evolved wood has a high perspective; these people are able to see the big picture, and they are the most compassionate humanitarians. There are two major emotional associations with wood:

- **Anger, frustration, and irritability**

- **Compassion, humanitarianism, and understanding**

The element of wood can be seen in facial diagnosis by looking at the structure of the forehead, eyebrows, and jaw. Wood is associated with the eyes, liver, gallbladder, tendons and sinews, and fingernails. A strong forehead, jaw, and brow bone indicate strength of wood in a person's constitution.

The eyebrows are a great place to look at liver health. If the eyebrows are weak and thin, then the liver might be overtaxed by toxins. I have frequently seen eyebrows fall out after an individual goes through chemotherapy, which indicates that the liver cannot handle the chemotherapy treatments; often, if you check labs, the liver enzymes will be elevated, indicating stress on the liver. The lateral third of the eyebrows are associated with the gallbladder, which relates to decision-making in Chinese medicine. If the hairs in lateral third are missing or extremely thin, the individual might be extremely indecisive, frequently changing their appointment times or having trouble choosing what to eat at a restaurant.

The fingernails are also a place to assess the strength of the liver. Weak, brittle, and cracked nails are a sign that the liver has been taxed by toxins or is constitutionally weak.

When wood is in balance, people sleep well at night and have goals and direction in life. They have roots, and they are well grounded. Healthy wood is strong yet flexible, like bamboo. Wood personalities are natural leaders. They are the most altruistic people. They have compassion for others, with an abundance of patience and kindness. Establishing charitable organizations and volunteering are activities that evolved wood people love. However, wood individuals can also be extremely competitive. For example, chess players often have a lot of wood characteristics. Wood people understand strategy. In Chinese medicine, the wood element is metaphorically related to the general of an army. Wood-dominant people tend to be athletic, with strong ropy muscles and visible sinews and tendons. They love athletic goals, such as finishing a marathon or triathlon. They relish debating and discussing politics.

One way I like to observe five-element characteristics is by analyzing clothing choices. Fashion—or even not caring about fashion—is a form a self-expression that allows a person's constitution to shine. Wood people appreciate designer labels. They like conservative clothing with a classic style, sometimes tending toward pretension. Often athletic with beautiful bodies, they might wear expensive athleisure attire.

Personality-wise, people with strong wood elements don't care if they pay full price for restaurant meals, personal services, clothing, or other goods as long as they are provided with superior service. In fact, strong wood element people often brag about the price they paid for an object.

Two organs are associated with wood:

- **The liver is associated with yin wood.**

- **The gallbladder is associated with yang wood.**

These two organs are the ones most affected by stress and frustration in Chinese medicine. The liver is associated with the uterus and menstruation as well as with the prostate. PMS, amenorrhea, endometriosis, painful menstruation, and recurrent miscarriages can be symptoms of liver imbalances. Prostate enlargement and prostate cancer are also reflections of liver disharmonies.

The liver also corresponds to the eyes. Visual problems are associated with liver pathology. Blurry vision, floaters, dry eyes, trouble focusing, myopia, and presbyopia are all symptoms of deficient liver energetics. Redness, itching, and broken blood vessels in the sclera are reflections of excess liver energy. But the liver is not just associated with physical vision; it is also about seeing the big picture and having goals in life—Condor vision!

The liver controls the tendons and sinews as well. I can often spot heavy metal toxicity because a client's body seems to have tendinitis all over. The liver meridian flows into the brain and ends at the top of the head at a point called Du-20, bai hui 白會, which means 100 convergences. This point correlates to the crown chakra at the location of the anterior fontanel. This is where we achieve energetic connection to the rest of the universe, allowing us to have an active relationship with the Divine. Because the liver travels through the brain, it plays an important role in memory, particularly memories of the past.

The gallbladder is the yang wood organ. Physiologically, it stores bile, helping us to digest fats. If bile cannot be released properly, problems digesting fatty foods might occur. Eating fats might trigger nausea, abdominal pain, and vomiting. Emotionally, the gallbladder gives us the courage to make decisions, allowing for decisive action. Gallbladder deficiency can lead to severe timidity and feeling discouraged in the face of mild obstacles. Gallbladder stagnation can be associated with deep resentment and bitterness about the past.

People with wood deficiencies might have multiple unfinished projects and have trouble focusing, with poor vision and an inability to visualize a future. Deficient wood can lead to muscle twitching, fasciculations, blurry vision, floaters in the eyes, headaches, and poor fingernail quality. In women, deficient liver energy can lead to amenorrhea or skipped menstrual cycles. If the liver channel is stagnant or blocked, a person might have problems connecting spiritually to a higher purpose (remember that the last point of the liver channel is the crown chakra). They might lack meaning in life, have a poor sense of personal purpose, and generally feel lost. People who are overly sentimental, who live in the past and ruminate over former experiences, often have a stagnant liver.

Treating the liver meridian can help them to move on so that they aren't stuck in the past.

Excess wood can lead to aggression, tyranny, anger management issues, and inflexibility. The inflexibility of chronic tendinitis is often associated with excess wood and long-standing frustration and anger. Chronic toxicity from heavy metals, mycotoxins, volatile solvents, and plastics can affect the liver, causing imbalances in the body that are reflected in the tendons, memory, vision, and sex hormones.

So, by looking at a person's forehead, jaw, eyebrow structure, tendons, and fingernails, you can assess the physical aspects of wood inside their body. Immediately upon looking at a client, I ask myself, What is the strength of the forehead and jaw? Does the brow bone jut out? Are the eyebrows thin or missing? Is the person dressed in an expensive suit or carrying a handbag that cost more than my car, flashing designer labels? What is their muscular definition like? Are their fingernails brittle and weak? Do they have chronic tendinitis? A lack of goals in life? Problems with insomnia? Issues with anger management or anger avoidance? I observe all of these things when assessing wood disharmonies.

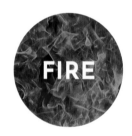

Fire is the most fun of all the elements. It is about passion, communication, and connection to the heart. Fire is associated with the South direction, the color red, passion, communication, and warmth. The archetypal image of fire is the sun. The sun represents the father in the sky who consistently rises each day, shining upon the Earth and generating warmth. In Paleolithic times, the campfire served as a place to gather in the evening and helped to keep people safe. Around the fire, they shared stories, cooked food, kept warm, and communicated information to their children. The fire element incorporates all of those things.

Think of a roaring fire. The flames naturally move upward and outward. Fire energy flames up and spreads and disperses, just as wood energy grows upward. Fire will burn what is above it and spread uncontrollably if not contained. It must be contained in order to be useful. One of the main problems I've observed with fire is that it can easily burn out. Fire people get bored! They are passionate and have a ton of great ideas, but they tend to jump from one project to another because they quickly become disinterested in what they are doing. Sustaining attention to complete a project can be a challenge for people with fire excess. Fire-type personalities are extremely social and like to do new things. They don't want to go to the same restaurant every week; they prefer to try one they haven't visited before! They often know about the newest, hottest trends and are ready to embrace them. Fire is the most innovative of all the elements.

Fire is about passion and joy. Fire types have a warm demeanor, and they tend to be creative and artistic. The flip side is anxiety. Imbalanced fire people have a tendency toward anxiety, just like wood people have a tendency toward irritability. Inappropriate or excessive laughter can be a sign of fire disharmonies.

In terms of clothing, fire personalities like bright colors and provocative cuts and tend to wear dramatic and asymmetrical attire. They often show hints of skin. Mixing and matching colors and prints is a fiery sign.

The element of fire can be assessed in facial diagnosis by looking at the tips of the facial features and cheekbones. When a client comes into my office, I look at the corners of the eyes and lips and the tip of the nose. Sharp, tapering, and distinct points indicate a plentiful fire element. Blunt tips or blurred edges of these facial features can indicate that fire is less plentiful. Curly hair is also a sign of fire.

Fire crackles and burns and is always moving. All of the fire meridians travel to the hands. People with plentiful fire often move their hands a lot while they speak, as the energy in the meridians of the hands is very active. Gesticulations and finger motions are expressions of fire energy. An inability to sit still is a visible sign of fire. Fire is about communication, and people with strong fire love to talk and are often excellent conversationalists. They enjoy cracking jokes and having fun. They can be dramatic and overly emotional.

The organs associated with fire are the heart, small intestines, pericardium, and san jiao (triple burner). All of the other elements have two organ systems, a yin-yang pair, with which they are associated, but fire has domain over four organ systems. I believe this is because fire is about the spark of life! The heart is considered the ruler in Chinese medicine, with all other organ systems being beneath the heart in the hierarchy. If your heart doesn't beat and you don't have that electrical spark of life with each heartbeat, then you cannot be alive. In Chinese medicine, the heart is metaphorically equated with the Emperor.

The circulatory system is also included in this association. Coronary artery disease, arterial plaques, peripheral vascular disease, and poor circulation are under the domain of fire. Looking at the tip of the nose is a good way to assess the quality of the heart and circulatory system. Redness indicates heat in the heart, which can be associated with anxiety, mental restlessness, palpitations, thirst, and insomnia. Dark red or purple veins on the tip of the nose indicate stasis in the heart and circulatory system, a diagnostic sign that the blood needs invigoration.

The small intestine is the yin organ to the yang of the heart. You absorb nutrients from your food in your small intestine. This is where your body discriminates between what to keep (good nutrients) and what to get rid of, sending the garbage to the large intestine to be formed into feces. That ability to know what is and is not good for you is a small intestine quality. People who cannot discriminate what they need to keep and what they need to get rid of in life have imbalances in the small intestine. In Chinese medicine, we say that the small intestine "separates the pure from the impure." This ability to discriminate, to know friend from foe, nutrients from garbage, is of the utmost importance in having correct barriers and the right relationship with the world. In the physical home environment, a lack of ability to discriminate can lead to keeping old broken junk, stained clothing, expired food, and useless items that can accumulate and cause clutter. In the body, IgG food sensitivities, leaky gut, and intestinal permeability are small intestine issues. Emotionally, people with small intestine disharmonies might have pathological relationships with toxic friends or family members, not understanding how to establish healthy boundaries. If the small intestine is in balance, we have the right relationship with what to retain and what to eliminate.

The pericardium is called the heart protector in Chinese medicine. Physically, it is a sheath of connective tissue that wraps around the heart. Metaphorically, the pericardium is like a secret service agent or ninja who acts as a bodyguard to the Emperor (the heart). People who have been hurt emotionally might have some restriction in the pericardium. This is an attempt to protect themselves from being hurt again. When the heart protector is working appropriately, those who would hurt us are kept out but those who are trustworthy, loving, and good are allowed into our hearts. People who have been wounded in love might have a tightening of the tissue around the tip of the nose, resulting in an emotionally constricted pericardium. This might be a clue for me to treat the pericardium channel so that the heart can be appropriately open to love.

The san jiao is the paired organ to the pericardium. San jiao translates as "triple burner." It is responsible for water metabolism in the body. This organ does not have a physical presence like the other organs in Chinese medicine. The san jiao is divided into three areas:

- The upper burner is located above the diaphragm.

- The middle burner is located between the diaphragm and the navel.

- The lower burner is located below the navel.

A traditional qi gong image of the san jiao is that each burner is a water wheel, moving fluids along in a steady manner. If the wheel gets jammed or clogged, fluids or phlegm can accumulate. So, if you have phlegm in your nose with a postnasal drip, you have a disharmony of the upper jiao. Fluids accumulating in your abdomen, such as ascites, is a middle jiao issue. Edema in your feet is a lower jiao issue. Urinary issues and chronic diarrhea or constipation can be viewed as lower jiao problems. Traditionally, the upper jiao is thought of as a mist, the middle jiao as a maceration cauldron, and the lower jiao as a drainage ditch.

The san jiao illustrates the relationship between fire and water in Chinese medicine. The fire of the san jiao is needed to metabolize water throughout the body. Too much fire and the fluids will be dried out and everything will be scorched. Too little fire and the fluids can flood the interstitial spaces, resulting in an overabundance of water with swelling and heaviness. A healthy san jiao helps us to keep our water metabolism in balance.

People who have excess fire tend to be dramatic, feeling extremely intense emotions. Often, after a few days or weeks, the emotion has burned out and they have a change of heart. This quick change does not mean that the emotions are not sincere. They are deeply felt, but because fire crackles, flames, and changes quickly, the emotions can run out of steam. Mania can be a type of excess fire. And mania eventually will wear out your neurotransmitters and cause you to crash, leading to depression and depletion. The intense fire of mania is not sustainable. Fire can easily burn itself out! If fire is deficient, the person will lack passion and joy. There will be a combination of restlessness and anhedonia. Burned-out fire has a sad and scorched quality. Balanced fire is consistent, like the sun rising every day. No matter what happened the day before, the sun will rise and shine on all creatures, good or bad. Balanced fire has a brightness and warmth that will generously be shared with others.

By looking at the tips of a person's facial features, their choice of clothing, and their hand movements, you can observe a lot about the quality of fire in their health. Do they gesticulate when they speak? Do they appear anxious or have a nervous tremor? Is the tip of their nose bright red, or are there multiple dark purple veins around the tip? Is their hair curly and messy? Is their clothing sexy and vibrant colored? Are they constantly moving, or are they able to stay still? Are they especially gregarious? A good communicator? Do they easily get bored? Do they want you to stay and entertain them during acupuncture treatments rather than have quiet, peaceful meditation time? Are they warm-hearted with a joyful demeanor, or have they lost the ability to feel joy? These are aspects that I consider when I'm analyzing the condition of the fire element.

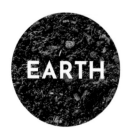

EARTH

Earth is the most comforting of all the elements. Earth nurtures us and helps us feel grounded and centered. It provides a home to all creatures. The Earth in Chinese medicine is associated with the color yellow, the organs of digestion, and the quality of the muscles. The spirit animal of earth is the Yellow Earthworm, turning over the soil and ensuring richness and healthy mineral content. The direction associated with earth energy is the Center, bringing us back to our sense of self and allowing us to feel grounded.

Earth can be assessed by looking at the quality and fullness of the cheeks, the size and shape of the lips, and the quality of the muscles. Wide, full lips are a sign of plentiful earth energy. Assessing the mouth is intrinsic to understanding the strength of the earth element because this is where nourishment begins. Digestion starts with mastication and the release of salivary enzymes that help to break down our food. The cheeks are another important place of assessment because you can see the muscles of mastication there. The Chinese believe that plump cheeks are a sign of healthy earth energy. Episodes of mass starvation and famine happened multiple times in China's history, so having access to plentiful healthy food is culturally important. Plump cheeks are called "moneybags" in Chinese culture. This does not mean that you are necessarily monetarily rich, but rich in earth energy and a sense of abundance. Sinking cheeks indicate inadequate resources and are a sign of depleted earth.

Earth people love to store things. They always have extra food, supplies, medications, and bedding and are willing to share with others in need. In a natural disaster, such as a hurricane or an earthquake, an earth person will have enough supplies to make it through. If earth is in balance, there is a sense of abundance.

Earth people are the most amiable of all the elements; even strangers feel comfortable in the presence of someone with earth abundance. They love to build social networks. They need to feel a sense of community. Earth people love to sit and relax. Comfort is extremely important to earth types. Often they have a special cushy chair. Many love to cook and put together large meals for friends and family, such as a Thanksgiving feast. Earth people can become overly concerned about trying to accommodate and please everyone, which can make them feel pulled in many directions. They are often the peacemakers in a family.

In regard to fashion, earth people value comfort over all else. They like snuggly and cozy cotton sweatsuits, loungewear, leggings, and socks. Cuteness is an earth quality as well; they might wear a t-shirt with a cartoon character on it. And because they love the idea of being part of a group, family, or community, having a photo taken of the family in matching outfits is the embodiment of earth ideals.

The spleen is the yin earth organ. In Western medicine, the spleen filters the blood, removing malformed and damaged red blood cells, and plays a large part in the immune system. However, the role of the spleen in Chinese medicine is more evocative of the pancreas in Western medicine. The pancreas is a gland that has two basic functions in Western medicine: it has an exocrine function, where it secretes pancreatic enzymes into the intestine via the pancreatic duct, and it has an endocrine function, releasing insulin so that glucose can be taken up into the muscle cells and brain. Insulin allows glucose to get inside muscle cells so that it can be used for energy. In Chinese medicine, the spleen energetically fulfills the functions of the Western medical pancreas. The spleen allows us to transform our food into basic constituents and then distributes those constituents throughout the body. We call these functions "transformation and transportation" or "TnT." The spleen accords us the ability to digest our food, just like the pancreas supports digestion by releasing exocrine digestive enzymes. These pancreatic enzymes break down food into amino acids (the building blocks of protein), essential fatty acids (the building blocks of fats), and carbohydrates (sugars), which can be easily absorbed. The spleen then transports the energy derived from food to the rest of the body.

Spleen qi deficient pathology is characterized by poor digestion with abdominal discomfort, bloating, central abdominal pudginess, loose stools with undigested food, and a tendency for fluids to accumulate in a pathological way. Diabetes is a type of damage to the earth element, which can occur from overconsumption of sweets. The earth controls water, and the spleen performs transformation and transportation. Think of a dam (earth) controlling the water flow of a river. If the earth element becomes weak, dampness can accumulate in the body because the spleen is not able to transform and transport fluids. Fluids accumulate, leading to dampness. Dampness can be mild, with just a swollen sensation and a feeling of internal heaviness, or it can become severe, with a lot of peripheral edema. If fluid sits for a long time without moving, it can lead to phlegm. The phlegm might manifest in the nasal passages, or it can come out in the stool as mucus. Phlegm and dampness indicate that the spleen is unable to perform the TnT functions adequately.

We have an aphorism in Chinese medicine that "the Spleen controls the four limbs." The "four limbs" refers to the arms and legs and the ability to move oneself in space. The spleen is what allows us to have mobility; it controls the muscles. This equates to how the pancreas helps glucose to get inside the muscles. Since the muscles are under the control of the spleen, one of the best tonics for the spleen is physical exercise. Deficiency of the spleen can lead to flabby and untoned muscles.

Another aphorism is "the Spleen banks the blood." The spleen is responsible for holding blood within the vasculature. So, if the spleen is deficient and energetically unable to hold the blood, easy bruising might occur, or a menstrual cycle might be extremely prolonged with heavy menses. The spleen qi has a rising aspect to it, so all prolapses are partially due to the Spleen qi sinking in the wrong direction. Hemorrhoids and uterine, bladder, and rectal prolapse are the result of the spleen being too weak to lift upward. Strengthening the energy of the spleen can help treat these medical issues.

The spleen is also responsible for "yi," which is translated as intellect. While the liver is involved with the memories of past experiences, the spleen governs working memory. Working memory allows us to store and manipulate temporary information and carry out complex cognitive tasks, such as reading, learning, and reasoning. The ability to memorize your social security number or a list of vocabulary words for a Spanish quiz is a function of the spleen. Being able to associate a new concept with previous ideas and remember and respond to information offered during a conversation are also spleen functions. Overusing the intellect can be taxing to the spleen. I often see students come into my clinic with extremely impoverished spleen energy. They are eating on the run, not exercising, and overusing memorization skills, a lifestyle that is not conducive to spleen health.

To have a healthy spleen, it is imperative to eat balanced meals in a comfortable setting at the same time each day so that blood glucose can be regulated and food can be digested under parasympathetic conditions. "Rest to digest" is a mantra of the spleen. If you are eating in your car as you drive through traffic to work, your spleen is going to be unhappy. Watching upsetting news on TV or arguing with a family member during a meal is another way to unbalance the spleen. Regular exercise strengthens the muscles and thus helps strengthen the spleen. Routine meditation time where you stop overthinking allows your mind to rest. This gives the intellectual aspect of the spleen a break, restoring the capacity of working memory. The spleen is the yin aspect of earth, and it needs daily circadian rhythmic support. Think of the daily rhythms of the earth, such as sunrise and sunset. The spleen likes to have a steady routine of meals, rest and relaxation, and exercise.

The stomach is the yang aspect of the earth. The Chinese medical aphorism is "the stomach rottens and ripens the food." Visualize your stomach acid breaking down your meal so that it can be more easily digested. The energy of the stomach is about decomposition and assimilation, breaking things into small bites so that they can be incorporated into the body's structure. Since earth energy relates to the intellect, the stomach is also about the ability to assimilate new information. The energy of the stomach can be stressed and impoverished by too many mental activities or family and social obligations—literally biting off more than you can chew. If you eat the correct amount of food, your appetite will be satiated and you will no longer be hungry. If you truly process information, you are able to retain it, integrate it, and make it accessible in your brain. My husband used to tease me about how I clenched my jaw as I studied and memorized massive amounts of information in conventional medical school and again in Chinese medicine school. My attempts to assimilate that information led to temporomandibular joint disorders (TMJ), which are a type of excess energy in the stomach meridian, as the stomach meridian travels through the muscles of the jaw. I have seen TMJ happen when people overextend themselves socially by caring for family members, volunteering at church, driving the kids to team sports, and baking for the school fundraiser. These earth activities are lovely things to do as long as you don't burn yourself out in the process. Having too many social obligations can burden the stomach, leading to excess stomach energy that manifests as worry, TMJ disorders, and acid reflux. People who have excess stomach energy might be chronically hungry and unable to feel satisfied after eating. They have an indeterminate gnawing hunger, yet they cannot figure out what to eat.

If earth is in excess, people may perseverate over problems. Obsessions, compulsions, and intrusive thoughts can occur if the earth element is overstrained. Concern for others can turn into meddling, clinginess, and overbearing attachments if the earth element is excess. Self-sacrifice or martyrdom is an excess earth action. A deficient earth element leads to social isolation, feelings of lack of abundance, and a lack of being grounded. Worry, overthinking, and too much intellectual work can injure the earth element, leading to digestive disorders, abdominal bloating, and poor muscle tone.

Facial analysis helps us to assess earth energy. Are the lips thin, cracked, and peeling, or are they plump and full? Are they extremely large in relation to the rest of the face? Are the cheeks plump like a baby's, or are they depleted, shallow, and sunken? What is the client's muscle tone like? Can you see tension in their jaw from across the room? Do they arrive late, rushing into the office because they have overextended themselves? Are they taking care of others and neglecting themselves? Are their ankles swollen and edematous with dampness? Is the central abdominal region plump, or are they extremely thin and malnourished-looking? Are they carrying around a bag of candy because they crave sweets? Have their muscles atrophied? Are they wearing loungewear? These are phenomena that I observe as I'm sizing up earth qualities.

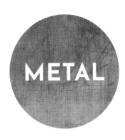

METAL

Metal is the element that is associated with the West direction, justice, fairness, integrity, beauty, art, refinement, logic, intellect, and intuition. It is about inspiration from heaven and standing in the light of your own truth. The West is the direction of the setting sun, which can be associated with death and dying. Autumn is symbolic of metal, and it is the time when the leaves fall from the trees onto the ground. The leaves get broken down into mulch, which nourishes the Earth. This is a time of decomposition and decay, with a downward descent. Several cultures hold ceremonies to honor dead ancestors in the Autumn. In traditional Chinese culture, fall is when the veils between the different dimensions of the world are thin. The energy of autumn facilitates communication with those who are in other dimensions.

Metal is interesting because it has a built-in dichotomy. There is downward movement, like leaves falling from trees, but there is also the energetic aspect of diffusing. The lungs and large intestines are associated with metal in Chinese medicine. Imagine drawing in a deep, refreshing, and energizing breath. You pull fresh oxygen into your body. This inhalation has a downward direction. But then the lungs help to diffuse this oxygen to the rest of your body, distributing it evenly. This fair distribution of diffused oxygen is another characteristic of the direction of metal. Metal has a downward and yet a diffusing direction. After taking a deep breath, you have to exhale. This is a way to expel toxins, keep pH balanced, and eliminate gases such as carbon dioxide.

The large intestine also allows us to let go of the things we don't need. Metal, being associated with the lungs and the large intestine, is about letting go mentally and emotionally and also about physical detoxification through exhalation, sweating, and defecation. The lungs control the skin in Chinese medicine, so sweating is the part of the detoxification process that is controlled by the metal element. The large intestine is responsible for defecation.

If we break down the concept of metal into even smaller parts, mitochondria are crucial components of metallic energy. Mitochondria perform cellular respiration, which is a set of metabolic reactions and processes that require oxygen. Cellular respiration allows energy from macronutrients to be turned into ATP, which is energetic currency. Mitochondrial health is a reflection of the health of the metal element in the body. Toxins can easily affect mitochondrial health, leading to impairment of cellular respiration, the accumulation of free radicals, and overall fatigue. Mitochondria are about the ability to utilize oxygen, a microsystem parallel to the lungs.

In Chinese medicine, the lungs are considered a delicate organ. They are susceptible to exterior pathogenic factors, which can include viruses, bacteria, fungi, air pollution, and etheric entities. The lungs are our initial boundary against the invasion of exterior pathogenic factors and our interface with the environment. According to Chinese medicine, environmental conditions, such as cold, heat, dampness, dryness, and wind, can invade and affect the body. People with metal disharmonies are often overly sensitive to environmental shifts and external stimuli. For example, a person with an imbalanced metal element might have a hard time sitting under a blowing air vent in a restaurant. They are naturally more affected by the environment and often have exquisite sensitivity to foods, air quality, and noise pollution. The skin of people with metal disharmonies is often quite delicate, easily becoming irritated and red. Allergies, whether environmental or food, are a sign that metal is imbalanced. People with strong metal qualities are often aware of environmental subtleties that other people might miss. Metallic people may pick up clues about how others are thinking and feeling, as their boundaries can be very thin. They might feel another person's emotional pain. They are often good at reading others, as intuition is a metal quality. There is a psychic aspect to people with a strong metal influence. The extreme emotional, physical, and psychic sensitivity to the environment can make it difficult for these individuals to cope with day-to-day reality. Because boundaries can be an issue, people with metal disharmonies are often especially sensitive to ghost-type energies and are more susceptible to acquisition of etheric entities, toxin accumulations, and parasites.

Metal has two aspects: a yin aspect, which is equated with jewelry, and a yang aspect, which is compared with a dagger or sword. Metal gains strength by being refined and forged in a fire.

Think of a jeweler sculpting a delicate piece of jewelry until it is exquisite, or a sword being hammered and placed into a fire over and over again until it is a perfect weapon. People with metal disharmonies often strive toward perfection and are constantly trying to refine themselves. If this element is unbalanced, the perfectionistic streak can become debilitating, resulting in not getting anything done because nothing is good enough. People with strong metal often have a self-critical side. They don't need criticism from other people because they are pushed by their own internal standards. They are often more interested in the process involved in accomplishing a goal than the goal itself. Metal is concerned with refinement, polishing, clarifying, and purifying until perfection is achieved. This is an internal process, and most metallic people crave time alone with a lot of personal space.

In the five-element cycle of phases, metal represents the movement of energy from Heaven downward. For example, various metallic ores are found deep within the Earth. Jeffrey Yuen taught me that metal represents the movement of the immaterial form into the material form. It is the energy of manifestation and concreteness. Crystals, metals, rocks, and gemstones found deep within the Earth illustrate this manifestation of form. The ultimate representation of metal is an asteroid falling through the atmosphere and landing on Earth. Imagine a large asteroid making a crater in the surface of the Earth; there is a dual aspect of downward and yet dispersing energies. Rare metals are frequently found in meteorites.

Lightning strikes are also a representation of metallic energy; they represent Heaven coming down to Earth and dispersing electricity. Ozone, which is generated by thunderstorms, contains three oxygen molecules that rapidly dissociate. Ozone is a metallic energy, as one of the major functions of metal is protection. Ozone's basic effect is to protect the Earth from the harmful effects of UV radiation. In medical ozone therapy, ozone can be generated with a special machine, and ozone's dynamic resonance structure can be used medically to facilitate physiological interactions that are useful in a variety of pathologies, including fatigue, toxicities, cancer, and chronic infections. I use ozone therapies in my clinic with the intent to activate metallic activities of protection, detoxification, and mitochondrial cellular respiration.

The nose is the main entrance to the lungs; it is where we draw in oxygen. So, to assess metal, we look at the nose. The larger, stronger, wider, and more prominent the nose is, the more metal is innate in a person's character. I learned from my mentor, the Master facial diagnostician Lillian Bridges, that if a person's nose sticks off the face by more than an inch, that person is a trailblazer and an innovator. The nose is "the money box of the face" where we draw energy from the atmosphere in the form of oxygen. Money, which is a form of energy, was traditionally made of metal coins. And the structure of the nose can be analyzed to assess the individual's ability to materialize and extract energy or save money. Another way to identify metallic facial features is to look at the spaces between features. Metal is about space, air, breath, the pause, the interstitial. Features might appear chiseled or precise. Highly symmetrical faces indicate the influence of metal as well. The secondary features of metal are the cheekbones, upper cheeks, and skin. The large intestine is shown in the lines between the nose and mouth, often called smile lines. In Chinese medicine, these lines represent purpose lines. The rim of the lower lip also reflects the health of the large intestine. The skin is the first line of defense and creates a boundary for the body. For this reason, it is a manifestation of metallic energy. In Chinese medicine, the lungs control the opening and closing of the pores, facilitating detoxification. Healthy metallic capacity leads to skin that is fine and smooth.

Beauty is an intrinsic aspect of life for metal people. They often are artistic or appreciate the arts. They acknowledge the fine qualities of objects and enjoy things that are well crafted. They are concerned more with the quality of an object than the cost or the designer label. Individuals with strong metallic streaks often have a refined sense of clothing style with particular attention to nontoxic, high-quality, natural luxury materials. Frequently, they wear delicate, intricate jewelry or accessories with metallic sheens. Often they find clothing tags irritating to their sensitive skin and need to cut the tags out. They might have a regal elegance and be conscious of their posture. They might appear aristocratic, and they are often well mannered.

Grieving and sorrow are emotions that can damage the lungs and large intestine. Long-term, unresolved depression will eventually deplete the normal Chinese medical physiologic activities of metal (breathing, sweating, and defecation). If metal is imbalanced, integrity can turn into hypocrisy. Structures can become overly rigid and uncompromising. Logic can turn into self-doubt. The restorative traits for metal are personal integrity, following your intuition, and attuning to your personal principles. When in balance, metal exudes a sense of integrity and fairness. People know where they stand with metallic individuals. Structure and control create an environment of equanimity, harmony, and serenity.

As I observe a client for metallic traits, I assess the nose and the spaces between features in terms of physiognomy. What is the rate and quality of the breath? Is the posture slumped and collapsed, or does the person have the posture of a ballet dancer? Are they well mannered? Do they exude boundary issues? Are they displaying symptoms of multiple chemical sensitivities? Do they require a clean environment or open space to feel comfortable? Do they need a lot of alone time? Are they intuitive or intellectual? Do they have chronic constipation or diarrhea? Asthma or COPD? Chronic infections? Are they unable to sweat despite intense cardio exercise? Do they have genetic impairments in detoxification? What is the quality of the skin? These are the conditions that I assess when evaluating metal in a client.

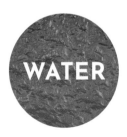

Water is associated with the North direction, winter, internal retreat, and the color black. The animal image of water in Chinese medicine is the black turtle. Water is linked to generative and regenerative forces; therefore, it is about procreation. Water is about internal stillness. In Chinese medicine, the water in the body is associated with the kidneys, bladder, brain and spinal cord, bones and bone marrow, reproductive organs, adrenal glands, lower back, hips, knees, teeth, and hair on the head. The ears and sound are associated with water. The North direction is associated with ancestral knowledge and the Big Dipper. In Taoism, the Big Dipper represents a place to which you can orient yourself; it allows you to have a compass in life, and it is associated with the center of the eight directions, the ba gua 八卦. Water takes the shape of any container in which it is placed, so it has an inherent capacity for adaptation. It also represents our inherent life force. In Chinese medicine, water is associated with the zhi 志, which is willpower. Water is the element that carries the jing 精 essence in Chinese medicine. Recall our previous discussion in regard to water as the corollary for the acupuncture meridians. Water is a conductor of sound and electricity (remember collagen and the piezoelectric effect) and a conduit for life itself.

Water has the capacity to dissolve a variety of molecules and substances—more than any other known substance—hence it is considered the universal solvent. Water's role as a solvent helps cells transport and use substances like oxygen and nutrients. That's why, as NASA scientists attempt to find extraterrestrial life, they look for evidence of water. Why is water such a crucial factor for life? In addition to being able to dissolve multiple chemicals, it is one of the few substances that can exist as a solid, liquid, or gas within a relatively narrow temperature range. It also has thermal properties that support life. Being a universal solvent, water can carry things into and out of a cell.

Water has a simple molecular configuration of two hydrogen atoms and one oxygen atom. The molecule has a bent structure, with both hydrogens tending to be located on the same side. This generates a partially positive charge around the hydrogen atoms and a partially negative charge around the oxygen atom. This gradient of charge, known as polarity, drives water's ability to be a universal solvent, allowing ions to be easily dissolved in water. A universal principle of chemistry is that opposites attract. Because water has both positive and negative poles, it is able to mix with and dissolve other molecules that are either positively or negatively charged. This means water intrinsically possesses fundamental and simultaneous yin and yang; each water molecule contains a dichotomy of forces.

When you put a bunch of water molecules together, they tend to line up so that the partially positive hydrogen atoms in one water molecule are attracted to the neighboring partially negative oxygen atoms of the next water molecule. This is called hydrogen bonding. The hydrogen bonds are strong enough to keep the water together and fluid, but weak enough to allow the water molecules to flow past one another. This hydrogen bonding generates the cohesive tendencies of water, seen with the fundamental surface tension of water. Watching an insect skim across the surface of water is a visible demonstration of water's ability to form hydrogen bonds that generate surface tension. So, water is fluid yet structured.

Water also has innate properties of adhesion, which is the attraction of molecules of one kind to molecules of another kind. Water likes to stick to itself, but under certain circumstances, it prefers to stick to other types of molecules, especially those bearing positive or negative charges. You might have seen water in a straw, where it seems to be slightly climbing up the walls of the straw, forming a meniscus (the water is lower in the middle and higher on the edges). These forces play important roles in capillary actions, such as for trees to move water from the roots to the leaves above or in the flow of liquids through blood vessels.

If you observe a water droplet, you are viewing the cohesion forces of water, holding it together. So, you have a good fluid environment combined with a universal solvent. Ice, as a solid, is less dense than liquid water. When a lake freezes, the ice is less dense and will rise to the top, leaving the heavier liquid water below the surface. This allows the microorganisms and other larger life forms within the water to sustain life. Water has a high specific heat capacity, which also makes it suitable for life. Specific heat is the amount of energy needed to raise 1 gram of water by 1 degree Celsius. Why does this matter for life? Many life forms can operate only within a certain temperature range. Because water has a high specific heat capacity, raising the temperature of 1 gram of water by 1 degree Celsius takes a lot of energy. This means that water has the ability to stabilize the temperature of the environment. Think of the temperatures within a single day in a hot, humid place, such as South Florida, compared to a dry desert, such as New Mexico. If you look at the daily temperature fluctuations, the places with a lot of water in the air will have much more stable temperatures after the sun goes down. In Florida, the high might be 89 degrees Fahrenheit and the low might be 82. But in the deserts of New Mexico, the high might be in the 90s and the low in the 50s. This lack of water in the air generates greater temperature swings. Water is a stabilizing force. It also has a high heat of vaporization. Evaporative cooling can take heat away from an organism so that it doesn't overheat. Water has a special ability to conduct energy and electricity, which is why you never want to drop a hair dryer into a bathtub full of water or go swimming during a lightning storm.

Winter, which is the season associated with water in Chinese medicine, is a time of internal retreat. This brings to mind animals that hibernate or slow down during the chilly months. Less sunlight is available, and the length of daylight is shorter, leading to alterations in circadian rhythms. People spend less time outdoors and more time at home doing sedentary activities, like reading next to a fireplace. Traditionally, winter is a time to cultivate stillness and retreat from the external world. Winter is a cycle of death in nature, which invites us to connect with the core of our inner being and deep untouched emotions. Increased need for sleep is common among all creatures as the days grow shorter. Sleep is an opportunity to dive into the element of water, as dreams are a way to vanish into the archetypes of the collective unconscious, allowing us access to creativity, ingenuity, and replenishment. Sleep and winter are times for consolidation, which the element of water encompasses. Consolidating means being very still and quiet and calling your energy back by doing nothing. This is the Taoist art of non-action, translated from the term *wu wei* 無為. Centering and collecting allows us to conserve, preserve, and regenerate our source energy.

People who have a strong water element are usually stable and wise and have the ability and courage to endure life's challenges. Strong introspective abilities and episodes of silence are common characteristics. The kidneys are the yin water organ, and the bladder is the yang organ associated with water. People with balanced water know how and when to filter something out of their body and energetic field. They wisely excrete toxins while maintaining intricate control of the balance of minerals within the body. They have a deep understanding of how to use their resources properly. Edema, renal insufficiency, and renal failure are reflections of water imbalances.

Since water represents our source energy, adrenal exhaustion is a type of Chinese medical kidney depletion. Physically, the adrenals are located on top of the kidneys, and they are included with the kidneys in Chinese medicine. Low DHEA hormone levels, chronic fatigue, and exhaustion are types of water depletion.

Water is also reflected in the reproductive organs, fertility, and creative force. A healthy libido, the ability to conceive if desired, and the ability to open up creative powers are signs of abundant water energy. Erectile dysfunction, premature ejaculation, low sperm count, low libido, irregular menstrual cycles, hormone deficiencies, recurrent miscarriages, and amenorrhea are signs of deficient water. Although fertility issues are often multifactorial, I find one common theme: long-term over-expenditure of energy, leading to jing 精 depletion. Writer's block and the inability to generate new works of art or harness creative forces are also forms of jing essence depletion. Creative forces can manifest in multiple ways. Jing represents our vital force; the ability to tap into jing is required for any generative process. Long courses of overwork, studying, sleep deprivation, and burning the candle at both ends can lead to depletion of the jing essence. Often, my clients who seek fertility enhancement are missing stillness in their life. Fertility of all types requires the ability to sit in incubation and wait for the spark of life to manifest. It requires patience and quiet, followed by a process of gestation and nourishment. Constantly being on the go does not allow new life to be nurtured. Yin activities of meditation, stillness, and reflection help to regenerate the jing force. The jing can be equated with the battery of the body, which needs to be recharged. This concept can be applied to physical fertility issues or can be extended to artistic endeavors.

Elementally, water constitutes our physical structure—bones and bone marrow. This concept of physical structure can be extended to DNA, which contains the blueprint for our physical structure and is inherited from our ancestors. Problems that involve bones, bone marrow, or DNA, such as osteopenia, osteoporosis, bone marrow dysplasias, leukemia, polycythemia vera, DNA damage, cancer, and single nucleotide polymorphisms, all represent damage to the water energies of the body. Deafness, hearing loss, and tinnitus are signs of kidney deficiency since the water element is associated with sound.

You can detect the strength of the water element by analyzing the face and observing the size and the strength of the ears, the area underneath the eyes, and the upper parts of the forehead and chin. Large, strong ears are associated with wisdom and the element of water. If you have seen statues of the Buddha or Confucius, you may recall their extraordinarily long earlobes, which represent wisdom, longevity, and plentiful life force. Strong chins can indicate plentiful willpower, zhi 志, and water life forces as well. People with large, robust chins can will themselves to live longer, even though their physical bodies might be deteriorating. A substantial chin can also indicate stubbornness, which is a positive trait when willpower is needed to overcome life-threatening events or illnesses. A client with a strong chin might actually be too stubborn to die. Dark circles under the eyes are an indication of a depletion of water resources. When I see dark circles, I know that the client needs a period of deep rest to allow for energy consolidation and restoration, as their essence has been exhausted. Loss of hair on the head demonstrates a weakening of kidney energy.

Water is associated with endurance, wisdom, and overcoming fear. Willpower is a strength of water. People with plentiful water might find themselves in situations that other people would not have the courage to endure. They might invest in huge financial projects or engage in risky activities like skydiving or race car driving. A deficiency of water can lead to debilitating fears, resulting in problems like phobias that can affect a person's ability to function.

Water people tend to be a bit sloppy about their fashion choices. Because water is associated with winter, sweaters and jackets exemplify water. Water people often choose black or dark blue clothing. Because they tend to be internally focused, many individuals with strong water are not concerned with their external appearance and just don't care about fashion. Of all the elements, they are the least sensitive to environmental influences.

As water people grow older, they often develop laissez-faire attitudes toward life. They tend to let things unfold and wait to see what happens rather than being active heroes. Because of this tendency, they can be viewed as lazy or indifferent. There is often an element of stubbornness in this attitude, but underneath, there is often a deep sense of peace and comfort with the state of the world as it is and a belief that everything has a purpose. There is a certain faith in the unfolding of life.

When a client enters my clinic, I start to internally analyze aspects related to water. What is the strength of the skeletal system? Is there a structural issue with alignment, like a hunched back? What are the size and qualities of the ears, chin, and the under-eye area? Does the person appear chronically exhausted from overwork? Are they quiet and introverted? Do they seem indifferent to the external environment? Do they radiate vitality and life force? These are the ideas going through my mind as I observe the element of water.

AUSCULTATION AND OLFACTION IN THE SERVICE OF DIAGNOSIS

I listen to the sound of a client's voice. Do they shout when they speak? Wood. Do they laugh inappropriately when stressed? Fire. Does the voice have a singing quality? Earth. Is there a sound of weeping, as though they are trying to hold back tears, or a slight catch in the throat? Metal. Is there a groaning quality to everything they say? Water.

INTERROGATION: THE ART OF QUESTIONING

Taking a medical history from a client is a necessary skill for any healthcare practitioner, and it's also an art. It tests both your ability to communicate and your knowledge of what to ask. This is a vital piece of the encounter with any client, and it can be pivotal in the healing process. Chinese medical school taught me a specific protocol for interviewing a patient, as did allopathic medical school. However, I find both of those methods rather limited, and I have evolved my own method of inquiry that is an amalgamation.

Often, clients come to my clinic after having been profoundly disappointed by conventional medicine. All healthcare practitioners want to help their patients. No doctor wants to hurt a patient physically or emotionally. However, because of high rates of physician and allied healthcare practitioner burnout, narrow paradigms of thought, insurance reimbursement–driven protocols, and limited time for visits, most of my clients have had a series of poor and frustrating interactions. They are often hypervigilant and feel hopeless, particularly in cases of chronic pain. Being present with someone who is in chronic pain and feeling irritable can be quite a challenge, and it requires some patience on my part and an opening of my heart.

There is also an art to achieving balanced empathy without feeding into pathological pity. Often in chronic illness, there are secondary gains, such as time off from work or avoidance of household chores. In the majority of cases, this secondary gain phenomenon is not generated via malingering or a factitious disorder but is truly subconscious. The pain is real. However, there are often deep unresolved attachments to wounds. I have seen multiple clients who have learned to define themselves by their illness, which can generate a detrimental sense of self. Others subconsciously use their illness to get attention from family members. As a healthcare provider, I strive to provide empathy without feeding into secondary gain. Taking a look at the possibilities of secondary gain can be an important step in the healing process. For example, a client might need to incorporate healthy ways to take time off from work to avoid burnout, like scheduled vacations, rather than feeling guilty about taking time off and pushing themselves to the point of collapse. This regaining of health is a process, a journey. I do not usually address these types of concerns initially, but once the client-practitioner relationship is solid and the client knows that I am truly concerned for their welfare, I may address aspects of secondary gain.

Having studied multiple modalities of medicine, including conventional medicine, Chinese medicine, herbalism, shamanism, functional medicine, medical astrology, and unrecognized illnesses such as mold toxicity and chronic Lyme and other infections, I have acquired the ability to hold multiple paradigms in my mind simultaneously. This allows me to have a wider perspective on pathophysiology as well as the ability to access a wide variety of treatment options.

When I obtain a medical history, my questioning is driven by a mixture of perspectives based on my knowledge from various studies. For example, when someone comes into my clinic for help with mental restlessness and mood stability and starts to describe a manic episode, I assess the situation using conventional DSM-V concepts along with Chinese medical patterns, functional medicine perspectives, and shamanic speculations. The diagnosis of the Chinese medical pattern "stomach heat" can consist of mental restlessness, insomnia, irritability, constant hunger with concomitant nausea or epigastric pain, and bleeding gums and is poetically known to include climbing to high places and singing. It can be interpreted as a type of mania. I might ask if the client has had any desire to climb to high places and sing. Often, when I ask, they are surprised at my question, but they answer affirmatively. This is not a question psychiatrists usually ask. From a functional medicine point of view, food allergies or infection with *H. pylori* might be factors contributing to this pattern as well. Often, the client has periodontal issues that need to be addressed, and I will refer them to a holistic dentist. Food allergies or parasites might need to be addressed in order to stabilize the mania, in addition to pharmaceutical help from a psychiatrist. From a shamanic perspective, the client might have intrusive energies that need to be removed.

Also, because I frequently see clients on a weekly or twice-weekly basis, we have more interaction time than would be expected for a standard medical or even a functional medical visit. A client's history unfolds little by little with each visit. Building rapport with a client can take time, as in any relationship. Often the client neglects to offer up important information until trust is well established.

I have a client who came to me for acupuncture help with debilitating migraines; these headaches had started when she was five years old. She told me that at age five, her headaches were so debilitating that her parents took her to Mass General Hospital in Boston, where she had a complete medical workup. At one point, the physicians even suspected a brain tumor, but the workup demonstrated no evidence of a tumor. She never received an adequate explanation for the etiology of her headaches, and she learned to live with them. She came for acupuncture regularly for two to three years, and the acupuncture did help reduce the severity of her headaches. Then, after all that time, she mentioned that as a small child, she lived within one mile of the Monsanto factory where Roundup/glyphosate was manufactured. She described the smell of the chemicals in the air. The timing of this exposure coincided with the start of her headaches. After this piece of medical history fell into place, we started doing some aggressive detoxification work, which enabled her to improve.

It is impossible to obtain every piece of vital health information that has occurred over a client's lifetime in an hour-long encounter. Sadly, toxic exposures are common. Noxious chemical exposures are frequently not in the consciousness of most clients. We as a culture have a certain cognitive dissonance about toxins and the roles they play in health. Recently, I went to a cancer center for my yearly mammography screening. Within the center of the building, they had a lovely garden called "The Healing Garden." I was wearing my shapeless patient gown and looking out the window, enjoying the plants, when a gardener wearing protective clothing came to spray pesticide on the plants. We know that most pesticides are carcinogens, but their use has become so commonplace that few people question it. Yes, it is common, but no, it is not normal. Toxins are a driving force in many common health problems, including hypertension, diabetes, and fatigue. Laboratory testing for these toxins is in its infancy, and most insurance policies will not cover labs that look at urine or blood levels of volatile organic solvents, pesticides, or plastics. Eliciting information about toxic exposures from a medical history can be difficult, as many clients don't think about it. Testing is not always feasible, as it can be cost-prohibitive and we do not have the ability to test for most of the chemicals in our environment to which patients are exposed.

As multiple medical modalities are respected, treatment options are expanded, allowing each client to choose what resonates best with them.

PALPATION

The act of palpation allows a lot of insight into the energetics of a client's body. Often, clients come in for acupuncture when they are in physical pain. Many of my clients have been to multiple physicians, chiropractors, and massage therapists before coming in for acupuncture. Some have been dismissed by their healthcare practitioners because their pain is not readily visible. Everything seems normal in a physical exam. Also, they are often experiencing sensations that they have difficulty describing.

I relate it to this experience: Recently, my car was acting up and making a bizarre sound. I took it to a mechanic and attempted to describe what was wrong, and I felt inarticulate. I lack a basic understanding of how cars work. And I felt utterly stupid as I attempted to describe what was happening. Luckily, I have an excellent and honest mechanic who was able to do some detective work based on my limited description. He found the problem and fixed my car. But as I stood there flummoxed, I realized that this is how many of my clients feel with they come into my clinic. They know something is wrong, but they have trouble expressing it as something concrete that a physician can understand.

When I begin palpation, I lightly touch the surface of the skin with my right index finger and middle finger. There is significance to the use of these two fingers. The tip of the index finger is where the large intestine channel begins, at an acupoint called LI-1. The large intestine is a metal organ, which is paired with the lungs in Chinese medicine. Metal is about inspiration from heaven, bringing information down from the atmosphere and into the Earth. The tip of the middle finger is the last point on the pericardium channel, called pericardium 9 or PC-9. The Chinese name of this point is zhong chong 中衝, which translates as "central chong." The Chong meridian is the deepest channel of the meridian system, traveling in the deepest center of the body. It is one of the Eight Extraordinary Vessels, which represent the body's innermost reservoirs. The Chong represents our bloodlines and ancestry, things we inherit from our parents and grandparents, going back several generations. By lightly running over the area of interest with these two fingers, I'm guided by heavenly influences (the index finger) and inner knowledge that goes straight to the heart and bloodlines (the middle finger). Using these two fingers allows palpation to occur with a balance of an inner intuition of the heart combined with divine guidance.

The physical force that is revealed to me as I lightly run my hand over the skin is the electromagnetic field of the fascia. To understand this principle, search the internet for simple children's experiments to explain static electricity. You can easily charge two pieces of Scotch tape with static electricity by placing one piece on top of the other (sticky side to smooth side) and then ripping them apart quickly. In the same way the charged pieces of tape can repel or attract one another, they will respond to your body's electromagnetic field if you hover the tape a few millimeters above your skin. The tape will dance in response to your body's electromagnetic fields, which run in the collagen. The tips of the fingers generate a much greater reaction to the tape, causing it to jump and dance. This is because a lot of electrical potential exists at the acupuncture points at the tips of the fingers and toes, called jing-well points. But, if you hover the tape along the course of an acupuncture meridian, it will waltz and shimmy in response to the qi of the channel. It is extremely subtle. You need to pay attention in order to feel it. But everyone is capable of sensing it. This is the sensation that I am palpating when I use my index and middle fingers on the skin. I am feeling for shifts in the electrical potential.

Sometimes, as I lightly run my fingers over an area of pain, I close my eyes, which allows me to focus the divine intuition (LI) and the heart protector (PC) in my fingers. My fingers glide over the area and automatically stop over the problem.

You can also sense if an energetic pattern is in excess or deficient as you run your fingers over acupuncture meridians. Sometimes there is a depression, which my fingers fall into. If the depression is deep, it can be like a vortex or black hole, sucking in energy. The client often feels a dull ache in this spot. The qi is deficient in these depressions. Other times, a lump in the fascia creates a small hill of congested energy. The excess qi has accumulated and gotten stuck there. These areas of excess tend to have more of a sharp shooting pain quality. Excess qi is treated with a dispersing technique to release the blockage, whereas in a deficient situation, the treatment consists of filling up the hole with qi in a tonification process.

As I glide my fingers, I also bring awareness to temperature changes. An area might feel ice-cold, like a glacier stuck inside the body. Other times, an area is hot, radiating inflammation. Sometimes the area of pain feels sticky, which indicates dampness. I often find that a combination of cold and dampness has penetrated a region of chronic pain. In Chinese medicine, it is believed that environmental influences and exterior pathogenic factors can penetrate the body, affecting the different layers within. The potential invaders include bacteria, viruses, and toxins but also climatic factors such as wind, cold, heat, dampness, and dryness.

In the Chinese medical diagnosis of pain, usually one or more climatic factors are involved: heat, cold, and/or dampness. Heat is a yang pathogen, which moves quickly and dissipates. It often burns itself out without intervention. For example, if you sprain your ankle, it will become red, swollen, and hot within hours. This is a form of damp heat in Chinese medicine. The swelling is dampness, and the redness and radiating hot sensation are considered aspects of heat. Weeks later, the heat will have dissipated and the redness will have disappeared. However, swelling might remain for months after a bad sprain. Dampness is a yin pathogen, which has a lingering quality.

Cold is also a yin pathogen. It is an extremely slow-moving energy that gets stuck. If you have an area of chronic pain and injury on your body, it is frequently a cold energy that is stuck in your body. You can palpate this on yourself. For example, I've had a chronic left piriformis injury since 2012. If I palpate my chest or abdomen, it feels warm and pleasant. But over the left piriformis, it feels like a block of ice. From a modern physics perspective, cold is simply the absence of heat and movement. However, in Chinese medicine, cold is a physical entity that can penetrate the body. This cold gets trapped in the wei 衛 level of the muscles. Cold sets up a physical blockage of the circulation of the wei qi 衛氣, preventing the sublimation of qi and suppressing the homeostatic abilities of the body. The wei level is the most exterior level of the body, which lies between the surface of the skin and the muscles, including the interstitial spaces and the fascia surrounding the muscles. The wei qi hovers at this level of the subcutaneous and interstitial region like an aura, protecting this layer. Wei qi is our first line of defense from interior invasion. It protects the body from all exterior pathogenic factors, including bacteria, viruses, toxins, and climatic factors. When cold combines with dampness and gets into the wei level, two yin climatic factors come together, leading to chronic pain. Many times this is expressed in clients whose pain worsens in cold and damp weather conditions. If a cold storm blows in with a lot of rain, I start getting calls from clients who have exacerbation of arthritic pain, which has a damp-cold quality. This exacerbation of pain drives many elderly people to move to southern Florida for the winter months.

Wei qi 衛氣 also controls the opening and closing of the pores. So, with chronic pain trapped at the wei 衛 level, sometimes the pores will be stuck open over an area of the body. You can see and palpate this, too. A person might have smooth skin all over but then have small bumps, like chicken skin, over an area of pathology. Often in chronic neck and shoulder pain, the pores on the upper back are stuck open, and tiny holes can be seen on the surface of the skin. This means that the wei qi is blocked and is unable to expel the pathogenic factor. The doors of the body are stuck ajar. It sometimes looks like a bunch of open pores without blackheads over the posterior neck and shoulders. The wei qi also controls the hairs on the surface of the skin. If someone tells you a scary story and you develop goosebumps, you have experienced an activation of the protective mechanism of the wei qi. It happens automatically when fear is triggered or danger is sensed. It is an important response to be aware of. Your wei qi is communicating a sense of jeopardy. Every time I have ignored this sensation, I have come to regret it.

I also look at the color of the area of pathology after I palpate it. Remember, the point is to assess the terroir of the whole acupuncture channel region. If cold is trapped, the area might have a slightly lighter discoloration. If heat is present, you might see redness and tiny papules. If dampness is present, you can have what is called "pitting edema" in conventional medicine. There is so much fluid in the interstitial spaces that when you press down, you leave an indentation in the skin. Although this can occur in any part of the body, pitting edema usually occurs in the lower legs, ankles, and feet. Remember, dampness is a yin pathogen that sinks downward. It has an associated heavy sensation as well. If an area has a lot of dampness, you can sense a viscous, agglutinative miasma when you hover your hand over it. The air feels thicker there.

If the cold is chronic, often there will be telangiectasias (purplish or bluish discoloration of the veins), small varicosities, and hyperpigmentation of the skin. This indicates that the pathology has gone to a deeper level than the wei qi 衛氣; it has become blood stasis. It is essential to use blood invigoration treatment methods to address blood stasis pain.

Clients are often is amazed at the precision with which I can palpate painful spots. It is a process of sensing the electromagnetic fields of the collagen in the fascia and evaluating the quality of the qi and the temperature, pores, and external surface of the skin.

CHOOSING A TREATMENT PLAN

Choosing a treatment plan can be a complicated process. It is imperative to assess a patient's elemental constitution in order to prescribe a tolerable treatment that will benefit the patient. Different elements gravitate toward different types of treatments. Five-element analysis is crucial for me to read the energetics of the patient and to prescribe the correct medical formulas for the presented disharmony.

Remember that we all have multiple elements inside of us. One or two elements might predominate. The elements interact with one another. Some elements support one another and are mutually enhancing, whereas others have contrasting characteristics that create internal juxtaposition. If someone has a lot of wood and metal characteristics, they probably will have a lot of internal strife due to these distinctly polar forces. I've seen a lot of clients who struggle to combine earth and wood elements within their personalities. Balancing these forces is an art. And I try to choose treatments wisely based on the energetics I perceive. Humans are complex creatures. Multiple dynamic forces come into play when treating the qi of the body.

Although I call myself an acupuncture physician, some of my clients do not get acupuncture. There are multiple ways to affect the acupuncture meridians in the body, and needling is only one modality. Clients with a strong metal aspect are often extremely sensitive; they find acupuncture quite painful and cannot tolerate it. They don't need more metal in the body. Metallic people usually do well with Earth-centered treatments, such as herbs and dietary therapies, or Water-type treatments, such as sound healing. (Sound is waves, just like those found in bodies of water.) The fire element is the most reactive of all. Fire personalities often need fewer needles inserted than other types. Overstimulating a fire person can create combustion and make things worse. Wood people, on the other hand, usually respond very well to acupuncture.

Earth and Water are the two most yin elements. They are more difficult to move, and generating a reaction can require more needles than in a fire or metal type. Imagine moving mud with a bulldozer. Mud is earth combined with water. It needs a much bigger push than sand, which is earth dried out by fire.

These are the treatments that I use in my clinic:

- **Acupuncture** is ultimately a Metallic treatment. You insert metal into the body in order to manipulate the collagen structures.

  > People with strong metal disharmonies often don't tolerate acupuncture.

  > Fire people need very little stimulation to move qi. Too much stimulation will result in combustion.

  > Wood people usually respond extremely well to acupuncture.

  > Earth and Water people need more needles and longer time with the needles in place to move qi due to their innate constitutions.

- **Stone and crystal therapy** combines Earth and Metal. Stones are the bones of the Earth, and you dig into the Earth to find metals and precious gems. I use crystal formations during acupuncture treatments, placing the crystals around the body in a grid structure that incorporates the acupuncture points, generating an electromagnetic field to rebalance the electrical potential of all collagen structures.

  > **Stones** are an extremely material medicine. They represent the Jing level of the Earth. The Jing level is the ultimate materialization. Quartz, one of the most common minerals, makes up about 12 percent of the land surface and about 20 percent of the Earth's crust. It is composed mostly of oxygen combined with silicon. Because quartz has some of the strongest piezoelectric potential effects, this soil composition helps to generate the electromagnetic fields of the Earth, which support life on this planet. Using stones in conjunction with acupuncture points can generate a new vibration at the immaterial level. This shift in the electromagnetic potential at the immaterial plane allows the transfiguration of the material form. If we drew a diagram, it would look like this:

CRYSTAL MATRIX		GENERATES A PIEZOELECTRIC EFFECT

WHICH TRIGGERS THE REVERSE PIEZOELECTRIC EFFECT		RESULTING IN A NEW VIBRATION, A NEW ELECTROMAGNETIC FIELD

WHICH GETS CONVERTED BACK TO A NEW STATE OF MATERIALIZATION.

- **Sound healing treatments,** such as Acutonics®, tuning forks, crystal bowls, Tibetan bowls, and sound meditations, are ultimately Water-based treatments. Sound is associated with Water in Chinese medicine, as the ears are the orifice of the Water element. Sound vibrates more quickly in water than in air. These treatments are excellent ways of moving water and stimulating the deep essence of the body. Acutonics is an integrated approach to health grounded in Chinese medicine, psychology, science, cosmological studies, and sound healing principles. This noninvasive methodology works with vibratory energy created through sound. The sounds of planetary bodies are brought into the clinical setting through the use of precision-calibrated tuning forks and hand chimes. The tuning forks are placed on acupuncture points, and the vibration travels through the entire acupuncture meridian, harmonizing the body. Jungian psychology and symbolism is an integral part of each tuning fork. There is healing symbolism behind the sun, moon, stars, and planets. These sounds trigger deep healing by evoking human subconscious archetypes. Sounds are layered over the patient as they lay on the treatment table.

- **Dietary therapy** is ultimately an Earth treatment because it addresses nourishment. Food comes from the Earth.

- **Herbal treatments** work on the Earth and Wood levels. Both elements are involved with growth. And the liver has to process any herbs that are taken into the body, just as the liver has to process pharmaceuticals. People with weak livers from a Chinese medicine perspective might not be able to tolerate herbal treatments. Conversely, if someone has a very strong liver, they might need a much larger dose of an herbal treatment.

- **Shamanic journeying** combines elements of Fire and Wood. Fire is the imagination, which is needed to create a shamanistic journey. Wood allows for visualization.

- **Blood ozonation** is a type of Metal treatment. Ozone is present after a thunderstorm when sparks of electricity cause oxygen in the air to form ozone. Ozone can be given to a patient by inserting an intravenous line, drawing blood out of the body, passing ozone through the blood, and delivering it back through the vein into the body. Wood individuals tend to do best with blood ozonation.

- **Biophoton therapies** involve applying a variety of medical devices to the body to deliver different frequencies of light. Light is a form of fire. Biophotons are electromagnetic waves in the optical range of the spectrum—meaning light. Light photons can be absorbed by the skin and can be beneficial to the treatment of a variety of conditions, such as fatigue and infections. Biophotons can also be delivered intravenously in the form of ultraviolet energy (just off the light spectrum).

- **Vitamin IV therapies** bypass the GI tract and deposit nutrients directly into the bloodstream. People who have a lot of digestive disorders, which might render them unable to absorb herbs or nutrients, may benefit strongly from IV therapies.

Dr. Rowe has given us a vivid, beautifully written glimpse into the profound understanding of energies developed over centuries by traditional Chinese medicine and how she incorporates these perceptions into her ability to diagnose and treat her patients.

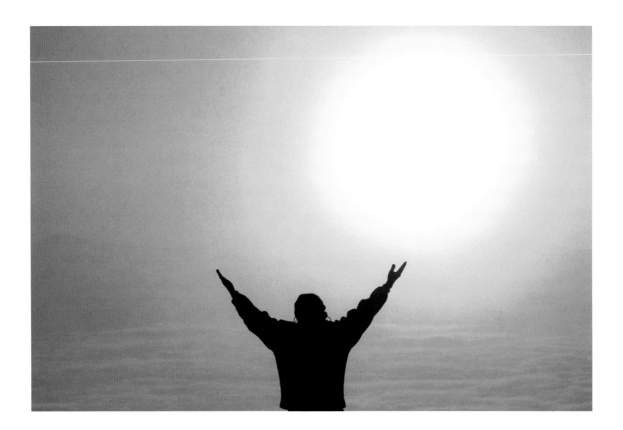

Emily Rowe, MD, AP, IFMCP, goes beyond the world of conventional medicine by combining intellect with intuition, holding multiple paradigms in her mind simultaneously. She graduated from the University of Miami Miller School of Medicine in 2004. After a brief time in the field of internal medicine at St Vincent's Hospital in New York City, she became frustrated with the Western approach to illness. She realized that she was being trained to treat the symptoms of disease and its end-stage complications while failing to address its root cause.

Inspired to find a comprehensive and definitive way to heal her patients, she went back to school and completed her master's degree in Chinese medicine and acupuncture in 2009.

She attended a class on Chinese medical dietary therapies with Jeffrey Yuen, a Chinese medical educator and 88th-generation Taoist healer, in 2009 at the Pacific Symposium in San Diego. Jeffrey Yuen has opened up higher levels of understanding over the past twelve years, helping her to evolve and cultivate understanding at multiple levels. In 2017, she again furthered her studies by obtaining her Functional Medicine Certification through the Institute for Functional Medicine. Dr. Rowe further advanced her education by studying Lyme disease and other tick-borne infections with Dr. Richard Horowitz and mold toxicity with Dr. Neil Nathan.

In 2018–2019, she attended classes with Lillian Bridges at the Lotus Institute and received her certification as a Master Chinese Medical facial diagnostician. This has enhanced her ability to work with the five elements from a Chinese medical perspective.

Dr. Rowe can be found practicing multiple modalities of medicine in amalgamation at the Miami Beach Comprehensive Wellness Center (www.miamibeachcwc.com).

CHAPTER 13:
Osteopathic Cranial Manipulation

One of the most profound ways of perceiving energy and its effects on the body can be accessed by the study of osteopathic cranial manipulation. There are several "schools" of cranial work, but from my perspective, the most effective was developed by osteopaths, led by the pioneering vision of William Garland Sutherland, DO. Almost singlehandedly, Dr. Sutherland put together an in-depth perception of the motion of the skull and the tissues within it.

I know that for many folks, even many physicians, the concept that the skull is capable of motion seems like a stretch. But Dr. Sutherland became aware of this motion, subtle as it is, and taught it to hundreds of physicians who learned how to use the information gleaned from his hands in the service of diagnosis and healing. For Dr. Sutherland, that perception of motion was just the beginning. Over the course of his long medical career, he recognized that there were more subtle energies that could be palpated, appreciated, and taught.

MY BACKGROUND IN OSTEOPATHIC CRANIAL MANIPULATION

From a personal perspective, I would like to recount my early experience with cranial treatments, which I describe in my previous book, *Toxic*.

My teacher of Reichian therapy, Phil Curcurutto, DC, encouraged me to go to Colorado Springs in the spring of 1975 to study this thing he called craniosacral treatment. At that time, I did not even know what an osteopath was; my medical school professors had told me that they were "like chiropractors." I quickly learned how wrong they were.

Prior to my first course in this field, I obtained a skull, and with the help of the book *Osteopathy in the Cranial Field* by Dr. Harold Magoun, I attempted to understand what I was about to pursue. It was clear on the first day of the course that, as an MD in a room full of DOs, I was a fish out of water. The fabulous faculty of osteopaths gave anatomical lectures that covered more material than I had ever been exposed to in medical school (even though I had been a teaching assistant in anatomy in my senior year of medical school) and then taught us how to feel the movement of the cranial bones. There are many cranial bones, and they do not fuse together completely as we age, as many MDs have been taught. After three eleven-hour days of trying to perceive this motion, I was frustrated when everyone else in the class, who had studied this technique in osteopathic medical school, appeared to be moving forward rapidly in their understanding. (I have often remarked that, knowing what I know now, I wish I had gone to osteopathic medical school so I could have learned basic medicine and osteopathic manipulation—a comment that surprises many people.)

At the end of the third day, Dr. Edna Lay, after allowing me to struggle a bit, put her hands over mine as I attempted to perceive these motions of the skull and guided me to a clear perception of what those bones were doing in the student I was evaluating on that treatment table. With her hands amplifying the motion that was present, I could finally feel this motion clearly. It was nothing short of a revelation—I got it. A whole world of perception opened up to me that day, and I will be eternally grateful to that entire faculty for taking me under their wing and showing me the art and science of osteopathic manipulation.

Upon my return home, I immediately applied what I had learned to successfully treat many patients whose headaches, neurological symptoms, and pains had baffled me before. Now, I could actually *feel* where their tissues were stuck, and I could restore motion and relieve pain using osteopathic cranial manipulation.

I continued to study with the Cranial Academy and the Sutherland Cranial Teaching Foundation, the two groups of physicians who provide this knowledge. Just when I thought I knew what I was doing with the bony structure of the skull, they gently showed me that osteopathic cranial manipulation was only the beginning. There are other perceptions of the movement of the cranial membranes, the cerebrospinal fluid, and the brain tissue itself that are equally useful perceptions (or perhaps more so). I spent years studying, learning, and improving those perceptions, which allowed me to provide better medical care to my patients.

Then, in the early 1990s, I had the good fortune of studying with James Jealous, DO, who was refining his understanding of Dr. Sutherland's teachings. Dr. Jealous developed what is now known as biodynamic osteopathy, which has added additional perceptual skills to the field of osteopathic cranial work, and allows for treatment on an even deeper level. These perceptions are so subtle that language begins to fail us as we try to convey what, exactly, we are feeling. To make it even more difficult, I have come to realize that practitioners process these perceptions through their own unique nervous systems, so we may all perceive the same imbalances but in different ways.

Biodynamic osteopathy is not the same as standard osteopathic manipulation in that it approaches treatment from a different perspective. In conventional osteopathic treatment, the practitioner carefully evaluates areas of blockage or dysfunction and then utilizes a variety of techniques to open those blockages and improve function. These are direct treatments of clearly perceived blockages. In biodynamic osteopathy, the goal is to open one's perception to the bigger picture. The obvious blockage may, in fact, reflect a compensation of that body to function better despite the blockage. The purpose of this compensation is to either protect another part of the body that is functioning poorly or to allow that part of the body to function better. Therefore, relieving that obstruction, or compensation, could take away the benefits of that compensation and make the patient worse. If we step back and "listen" with our finely honed perceptual skills, that body will "talk" to us and "show" us which area and tissues need to be addressed, and we can very gently "nudge" the body, using our own barely perceptible forces, to "move" in the direction of healing.

JEFF GREENFIELD ON OSTEOPATHIC TREATMENT

I'll let Jeffrey Greenfield, DO, take it from here with his description of a treatment for one of his patients, in which he helps us understand how these perceptions can enable a skilled osteopath to directly feel the connection between structure and emotion.

by JEFFREY GREENFIELD, DO

Sue was on my treatment table, the osteopathic treatment was nearly finished, and my hands were on her head; her scalp, cranial bones, dural membranes, cerebrospinal fluid, brain, spinal cord, sacrum and coccyx, hips, shoulders, feet and arms were all lined up; they felt unified as one "Whole." Her system was ready, idling, waiting for something big to happen. When we are able to get a patient to this point, health usually flows right in—but in this case it did not. Something was off or missing; the tissue, fluid, and fulcrums were all perfectly aligned, but it was not happening.

Sue had come to see me at the request of one of my colleagues. She had sustained a concussion several days before. She had fallen on her buttock and then flipped backward and hit her head. Although she did not lose consciousness, right after the incident she was quite disoriented. She had concussion symptoms such as fogginess, headache, and sound and light sensitivity. My colleague, also a cranial osteopath, treated her almost immediately and then put her on a concussion protocol with various herbal treatments, medications, and a special diet. He gave her a second osteopathic treatment a day or two later, and they both noticed she was much improved following that immediate intervention. However, she was still not back to baseline.

She came to see me about four days after the initial incident. She was still experiencing headaches and having difficulty concentrating, but the two treatments and the integrative concussion protocol had helped a great deal. Because of the fall, she still had significant back pain and neck aches. She noted that she was not quite back to normal.

I was familiar with Sue because I had treated her before. On my examination, I could tell that she was not quite herself. There were things that still needed to be addressed. One of the first things that jumped out at me was that her hips were unbalanced and her sacrum [the triangular bone that sits between the big hip bones in the lower back, just below the lumbar vertebrae] was twisted. In the cranial concept of osteopathy, if the sacrum cannot move, then the head (or cranium) may not be free to move because there is a direct and indirect connection between those areas. I treated her sacrum-pelvis complex (the pelvic bowl), allowing for freer motion.

As I waited for her body's innate healing mechanisms to kick in, I recalled that in past treatments, I had freed up this key issue as well as others, but the treatment would not "finish." Sue had recently told me that her father had died suddenly. As I was holding her tissues with everything lined up, I began thinking about a passage that my late friend and colleague Jayne Alexander, DO, wrote about loss on page 144 of the second edition of the *Textbook of Functional Medicine*:

Loss, in the context of trauma, is unique. Unlike other forms of trauma in which the integrity of the organism is disrupted by an added force…, in loss, [it] is disrupted by virtue of absence…in loss there may be an actual perceived absence in an aspect of the fluid field….

Here was the missing piece! I began thinking about her father with respect to this "absence" or gap that I felt. That was it. It was like I felt the essence of her father fill the room and allow the space inside Sue to fill. Everything was now lined up, and finally there was a spark—a light came on inside the third ventricle of her brain and penetrated all of her tissues, vivifying her fluids and her essence. She took a deep breath, and the treatment was over. The trauma of the concussion she had experienced was finally healing, as was the trauma of her loss, and now her tissues were able to work toward healing with no additional impediments.

Dr. Greenfield adds:

This is the essence of osteopathy, specifically cranial osteopathic treatment. This modality works to restore the health of a system. It involves knowing the minutiae of anatomy and physiology and linking them with processes that are inherent in nature. It involves honing perceptual skills, integrating them with medical knowledge, and applying principles of treatment with deep trust that those principles will lead toward health.

Although the science and art of osteopathy has been around for over 100 years, I discover new things every day. Every patient is different, and the same patient is different every day. Every treatment is an adventure, but some are spectacular and stand out, as did the case above and a case to be brought up later in this chapter. I am still an explorer. We osteopaths explore phenomena that occur in our relationship with life, health, and disease. We explore the "feel" of health, disease, and trauma and the integration of wholeness and loss; we are always looking for the feel of health.

Evaluation and treatment using osteopathy in the cranial field differs significantly in that it is not focused on finding and treating stuck places or "lesions," but rather on looking at the wholeness of motion and allowing the patient's body to reveal what needs to be treated first by careful "listening" with all of our senses using our hands as the focal point of perception. A cranial osteopath most often observes the inherent movement in a patient, trying not to interfere with it or add force. The inherent motion is a physiological process that pushes through the anatomy. In any given region of the body, the effects of primary respiration can move freely or not, thus revealing areas of health and areas of restriction without requiring the practitioner (or "operator") to use palpation or introduce movement into the system. The term "primary respiration" does not refer to breathing through the lungs, but rather the expansion and contraction of the tissues in response to what is referred to as the "cranial mechanism," which is innate movement of the skull as reflected by motion of the bones, dura, cerebral spinal fluid, and deeper energies to which Dr. Greenfield and I are alluding. The quality of movement and other characteristics give the operator information on the health of the entire person.

Dr. Greenfield adds to my description of this process:

The mechanical model is just that: We look for motion and patterns in the bones, joints, and fascia and often introduce a specific manual operation to reduce the problem. In the functional model, with the same pattern noted, the system is placed in a position of balance so that the tensions of what the operator feels in their hands are equal. This promotes a release by the innate motion already present in those tissues. Essentially, given the opportunity, the body heals itself.

The biodynamic model of cranial osteopathy (biodynamics) takes a little more explaining. As far as I am concerned, it is one of the most amazing tools I have had the opportunity to learn in osteopathy and in all of medicine, for that matter. The diagnostic and therapeutic potential is seemingly limitless—limited only by the operator's perceptual and interpretive skills. And given the diagnostic potential, it can clue us in to pre-disease states from inflammation, illnesses from viruses, Lyme and other tick-borne diseases (TBDs), adrenal fatigue, electrolyte imbalance, loss or death of a loved one, and many other stressors with which our patients have to cope.

If that sounds preposterous to you, it did to me, too. In my first year of osteopathic medical school—mine was the last of the original four classes in this new school—a local Maine osteopath was asked to help out in our Principals and Practice lab since he was so good at it. One of my friends and fellow students came up to me toward the end of a class looking quite loopy. He told me he had just gotten treated by a visiting DO who was able to chronicle many of his old injuries and traumas by region and the approximate time they occurred—"and…he floated me into space…." That visiting DO was James Jealous (who, as previously noted, developed the Biodynamic model of Cranial Osteopathy). My friend's treatment by Dr. Jealous was so profound for him that he came and grabbed me afterward to meet this visiting doctor, saying that this DO had gently put his hands on different regions of his body and was able to describe an accurate health and injury history as well as help resolve those injuries using very little force or movement.

As we all know, we have many types of tissue in our bodies. We have skin, organs, fat, brain tissue, bone, blood vessels, peripheral nerves, and much more. Each of these tissues has a slightly different feel to a trained operator. But when tissue is in motion, it feels much different than the other perceptions we are discussing. So all tissue has a similar field when compared to the perception of fluid or potency. We would refer to this, therefore, as the "feel" of tissues.

Similarly, there are many fluids in our bodies. We have blood, intracellular fluid, extracellular fluid, cerebrospinal fluid, and even fluid inside the bone matrices. Each of these fluids has a slightly different feel to a trained operator. However, they all have a similar feel when compared to the other effects of primary respiration. Tissue in general has more of a hydraulic force feel. Accordingly, we would refer to this as the "feel" of fluids.

The last effect of primary respiration to be discussed is one of the more difficult to describe. It is called potency. Potency is responsible for the vivification of fluid and tissue. When something is infused with potency, the feel of it can vary from something similar to an overcooked noodle (an inanimate, dull feel) to something extremely animated (shining and alive). Potency augments the tissue and fluid movement and penetrates them but is not really a part of them.

There are different types of potency that can be perceived. Sometimes potency moves in one direction, which is a vectorial potency. Other times it has an electric feel of what the resting potential is doing between cells and nerves in their environment. It can have a soft feel, like soap bubbles rising up through the tissue. Dr. Sutherland (introduced at the beginning of this chapter) has described it as the light of a lighthouse shining into the water. The light is in the water but not of the water. He has also related it to sheet lightning. This perception can be difficult to describe, but the bottom line is that potency can be perceived. Although various forms of potency can be distinguished, in general they have a similar feel when compared to tissue or fluid movement. I hope you are getting a sense of both how subtle these perceptions can be and how many important physiological processes we are capable of palpating and perceiving.

Other perceptual properties, not as well cataloged, occur in the system. As mentioned earlier in this chapter, I had pooh-poohed one of my teacher's statements that we can detect things like illnesses from viruses and electrolyte imbalances in a person's system using only our hands. With foot in mouth, I now know I was incorrect. Our sensory system can perceive things that continue to surprise me. For instance, when I started my practice, Lyme disease was not a significant illness in my area. As time went on, however, it became epidemic in my patients.

Dr. Greenfield will now describe particular perceptions that have been of unusual value in helping us diagnose and treat Lyme disease and mold toxicity in our patients. Spoiler alert: Dr. Greenfield and I have taught dozens of physicians to utilize what he is about to describe to improve treatments for the most complicated patients suffering with Lyme disease and its coinfections.

I developed quite a reputation for successfully treating people with unusual and even bizarre symptoms that would cause other practitioners to roll their eyes. Many know that Lyme disease and other tick-borne diseases cause unusual symptoms that are not currently alluded to in most medical texts. Around the year 2000, I started seeing a number of patients with these unusual symptoms. I noticed during treatment that they had an unusual "buzzing" I could feel with my hands. It felt like someone was banging on the black keys of a piano near middle C—a discordant, nonharmonic medium-frequency vibration in the tissue and the fluid.

I questioned the validity of my senses, because I soon felt this buzzing in a significant number of other people, and I thought it was a problem with my perception. One of my patients helped me realize that what I was feeling was really there. She worked with horses, which are prone to tick bites and Lyme disease. She was a specialist in equine massage. With certain horses, she began noticing a "buzzing" feel in their tissues. Most of them were not in tip-top shape and were not doing well healthwise. She thought they might have Lyme disease but was unsure. After several lengthy conversations, we agreed that we were feeling the same thing. We realized that the horses with the "buzz" that she was treating and the patients with the "buzz" that I was seeing all had Lyme disease or other tick-borne diseases (TBDs). Lab testing and other practitioners have helped verify what I and others feel in TBDs.

It appears that the majority of TBD patients have a certain feel to them, with a perceptible non-harmonic vibration. Often we can distinguish them, but the diseases and vibrations are overlaid on each other. Some of us are able to ferret out the various vibrational signatures by using herbal filters designed to treat certain tick-borne diseases. This gives us an idea of what to test for, where to start treatment, and how a particular treatment may be progressing.

We often find that when we treat a patient with a complicated illness (meaning an illness triggered by chronic inflammation, such as Lyme disease, mold toxicity, Alzheimer's disease, Parkinson's disease, or autism), our patient may have a positive response to treatment in the office but come back in a week or two having reverted to their pre-treatment state on both exam and symptom review. In other words, the treatment doesn't "stick."

When a patient gets to a certain point, we can figuratively reboot their system. In the language of cranial osteopathy, we call this process Ignition. I previously explained how a doctor can perceive motion in the tissues, fluid, and potency and how each of those has a distinguishing feel. In healthy people, these have different rates of fluctuation or movement but are in a harmonic dance with one another. These effects are also integrated with the Whole. This is not the case in those with chronic illness. However, when we have chipped away enough at the problem, improving the expression of health, an amazing leap can occur.

My patient Rachel was a forty-year-old professional in charge of a clinic. Her responsibilities included managing and working with the staff. She had been treated for Lyme, *Bartonella* (a Lyme disease coinfection), adrenal fatigue, and other manifestations of TBD. She had mold and mycotoxin exposure but had not yet been evaluated or treated for it. She was quite ill at the start of our doctor-patient relationship, but she had recovered greatly from her original condition. Some very skilled physicians had appropriately treated her for her conditions, and she thought she felt well. She was still on herbal treatment for *Bartonella*.

Rachel was familiar with cranial osteopathy and had gotten occasional treatments from other local osteopathic doctors. She came to me for osteopathic treatment knowing that I had a great deal of experience in treating those with TBDs using conventional, alternative, and osteopathic approaches. Her conventional physical exam was quite normal, but the evaluation using a biodynamic model of cranial osteopathy was not. Her tissue movement was present, but the force of fluctuation was diminished and a bit disorganized. The fluid fluctuation of her mechanism was present but was weak and lacked vitality, and it was not as connected with her tissue as it should have been. The feel of her potency was scattered. She had a slight medium-frequency vibration, but it was in the background, so I interpreted it to be a partially treated TBD.

I followed principles of treatment that are too involved to discuss here. Toward the end of the session, I was working to balance all of the effect, pulls, pushes, and movement from the head (cranial osteopathy). As I connected with the feel of the natural world around us that is in us but not us, I let her system be part of that. What happened next exemplifies the beauty of osteopathy and the privilege of being present for some incredible transformations.

With a small portion of my attention, I noticed the tissue fluctuation, fluid fluctuation, and feel of the potency go out like a low tide. There was a long pause in all motions. Then, in the center of Rachel's brain, likely in a structure we call the third ventricle, there was a spark, a light, some heat. It felt like a pilot light going on—the health was beginning to really show. Then a spark ignited the fluid, tissue, and potency with a feel of life, health, well-being—this was Ignition! The tissues, fluid, and potency were all now vivified, in harmony, working together and connected. Rachel took a long, slow, deep breath, and the treatment was over.

In her next visit, Rachel related to me that after that treatment, she came out of a fog that she had not realized she'd been in. Her thinking was clearer and her mind was working better. She noticed that she had been neglecting many of the finer details of her job responsibilities, but she was now able to spot those oversights and correct them. She felt awakened and refreshed. She knew she still had *Bartonella* and maybe mold, but she was feeling healthy again. Her system had rebooted. She continues to do well and gets regular treatments that hold, and her Ignition stays on.

JOEL FRIEDMAN ON CRANIAL MANIPULATION

To add to our understanding of this kind of perception, Joel Friedman, MD, one of my oldest friends and colleagues, will relate a story about his experience with cranial manipulation. Dr. Friedman has been studying and practicing this discipline for over thirty years and in the course of this treatment had this miraculous experience.

by JOEL FRIEDMAN, MD

Matthew's appearance in the doorway of my outdoor office startled me. Trying to act as nonchalant as possible, like I saw this sort of thing every day, I invited him in. I could not avoid staring at his face; one eye was situated below the other and sunken into his skull. It was down and back, the result of falling from a ladder and hitting his cheek on a branch on the way down. Not surprisingly, he had double vision, and his wife had driven him to my office from Hana (Hawaii)—a good two-hour drive.

These were new people to me, and as I sat and listened to Matthew's story, I wondered why they had come to me. I asked him, and he simply said, "I was told that you could help me." I explained that he had a "blowout fracture" of his orbit and that because of this fracture, the eye had lost its floor. He would need to go to the ER, and an ENT would need to do surgery to repair his orbital floor. He looked at me with his distorted gaze, and it seemed like nothing I said was getting through. I went on repeating myself and added that my training as a humble GP offered nothing other than to recognize the problem and perform triage. I slowed my speech, thinking that there may be a comprehension issue at hand. Matthew repeated, "I was told that you could help me." I said that by telling him to go to the ER and get this problem dealt with surgically, I was helping him. No matter what words I used or how I expressed myself, however, he would not leave.

I became annoyed. I thought, "What idiot told him that I could help? Why would he refuse to leave?" Soon, though, I realized that something deeper was at play, and I began to have an inner dialogue with whomever or whatever energy was behind this unfolding drama; I thought of it as God. The dialogue went something like this:

"Okay, God. I get that you brought Matthew here to me. I also get that, you being omniscient and all, you know I have no clue how to help this man. The way I figure, one of two things is going on: Either you have brought Matthew here for me to try to help him, knowing that I will fall flat on my face, this being one way that you entertain yourself. Who am I to deny your pleasures? But, if you brought him here for real healing, you'd best send me some help…something or someone who actually knows what they are doing."

I asked Matthew to lie faceup on my exam table. I was trained in cranial osteopathy and have been practicing diligently for thirty years. Still, no one had ever spoken of healing fractures with "hands-on" work, not even my teacher, Robert C. Fulford, DO, one of the pioneers of alternative medicine using osteopathy in the cranial field. I encircled Matthew's injured orbit with my four fingertips, making very gentle contact. I figured I'd fumble around for ten minutes or so and, after failing to help, send him to the ER. Not having a clue how to proceed, I went into a meditative state—a state I have always thought of as theta wave dominance. It feels like a state between sleep and wakefulness. In my experience, good things happen in theta.

In this somewhat altered but familiar state (I have had many years of practice cultivating more extended theta states; they are usually fleeting), I began to notice what felt like movements in my fingertips. The movements seemed to have a very specific ordered pattern, something I had never experienced before.

As an observer, I witnessed an energy that was clearly not mine coursing through me and into the fractured orbit beneath my fingertips. I would guess that this went on for five minutes or so. Then it stopped. I waited for Act Two, but none was forthcoming. After several minutes, I realized that whatever had happened was over, and I needed to return to normal wakefulness and open my eyes. I thought one of two things had just happened: either I'd just had one of humankind's grandest episodes of delusion on record, or something had actually changed, which was unlikely.

Something had happened. When I looked at Matthew's face, I saw that his eye was once again anatomically positioned in its orbit. It was normal in every way, and symmetry had been restored. His double vision was gone, and he could see perfectly. We had witnessed an instantaneous healing of a facial fracture. I was stunned; deeply moved and grateful, but stunned. Out of my mouth came words that have never been in my lexicon. I said, "Matthew, you have just been visited by the Holy Spirit, and you are 100 percent healed." And he was. He rose from the table, shook my hand, and walked out the door. I have not seen him or heard from him since, but I hear that he is still around doing his work as an arborist—more cautiously, I hope.

The thought of accepting payment for such a healing was out of the question. The experience severely rattled my cage and expanded my mind and heart over the notion of what is possible. So many questions flooded my mind, and so few answers were forthcoming. What exactly was this energy that had come from outside of me, and where had it come from? Was it a what or a who? And what could I do to make it come more often, as there are so many people who need this kind of healing? Why me, why Matthew, and why now? If such seemingly miraculous healing can occur, why had it not happened before in my thirty years of practice? Why is this sort of healing not commonplace?

On and on the questions came, and of course, I still have no answers. However, I now know that profound, even miraculous healing can happen and that it can come through me (and I suppose for all sincere healers). I must be present and have the intent to heal, but it is not me doing the healing. When I think that the healing will come through me and my skills, the results will be modest.

There is a need to be very present and then get out of the way so that this external source or presence can come through and effectuate deep healing. The results are beyond my control, and this is a big relief. As long as I believe it is me and my knowledge or skills that determine the outcome, I live in a perennial state of anxiety. Will I fail or succeed? Or worse, will I harm my patient? Do I know enough, or is my learning insufficient for the case at hand?

I now know that the phenomenon of healing is essentially mysterious. We often delude ourselves into thinking that we understand how healing occurs, but with just a little digging and humility, we see that we know very little when we are expected to know it all. Somehow, we must humble ourselves and gratefully embrace this glorious mystery.

I hope that Dr. Greenfield, Dr. Friedman, and I have been able to give you some idea of the breadth and depth of this method of perception. These motions that we are tuning in to reflect the energies that these tissues embody. With enough study and practice, we have learned how to tune in to this motion/energy of the cranial bones, the ligaments that tie these bones together, the brain itself, the cerebral spinal fluid, and, on even deeper levels, the biochemistry of these tissues collectively referred to as the "fluid body." At a deeper level, we can begin to perceive the "Ignition system" (which Dr. Greenfield alluded to earlier). This allows us to feel whether there is enough energy at the patient's core to energize the process of healing and allowing the tissues to come back into balance. A practitioner can perceive all of these things by gently and respectfully placing hands on a patient's head (or any other part of the body) and allowing these energies to make themselves known.

Joel Friedman, MD, graduated from the University of Miami School of Medicine in 1980. He has been in general practice for forty years. He can be reached at friedman@maui.net.

Jeffrey Greenfield, DO, describes himself as a hands-on osteopath practicing traditional cranial osteopathy. He has trained with mentors with direct lineage to study with Dr. A. T. Still, the visionary who developed osteopathy in the 1800s, including James Jealous, DO, the osteopath responsible for the biodynamic approach to osteopathy in the cranial field; Lou Hasbrouck, DO, mentor and friend when he was in the USAF; and Anne L. Wales, DO, a student of William Sutherland, DO, the developer of the cranial concept of osteopathy, who was himself a student of the first osteopath, Dr. Still.

Dr. Greenfield completed his osteopathic education at the New England College of Osteopathic Medicine (NECOM) and was a family medicine resident in an Air Force hospital in Florida and then an associate professor of family medicine at the Offutt AFB-University of Nebraska combined FM residency program. After separating from the military, he moved to New Hampshire and eventually set up his own osteopathic practice. After honing his treatment skills for those with chronic complex illnesses, he received an invitation to join the Gordon Medical Center to work directly with Dr. Nathan, Dr. Eric Gordon, and other top people in the field of complex illnesses. He developed a course for those trained in osteopathic treatment, *Detour of the Minnow* (a play on lectures by Dr. Sutherland called "Tour of the Minnow"), to teach physicians how to feel the energies of Lyme disease and mold toxicity. Several years later, he moved to Maine, where he continues to refine his abilities in working with patients who present with complex medical illnesses.

Practice Information:
Jeffrey Greenfield, DO
Osteopathic Healthcare of Maine
Osteopathichealthcareofmaine.com
98 Clearwater Dr.
Falmouth, ME 04105
207-781-7900

CHAPTER 14:
The Energies of Dreaming

I am told that my brother Gene and I look alike—enough that we have been mistaken for each other at medical meetings. Attendees sometimes come up to me and begin a conversation, and eventually it dawns on me that they were intending to talk to Gene. He has had similar experiences. He sometimes jokes that we are "twins born five years apart." Like me, he is an experienced medical clinician who has spent years studying integrative medicine and incorporating it into his medical practice. So I was delighted when he agreed to write this chapter, for which he has had some unique training, as you will see.

by GENE NATHAN, MD

We spend somewhere around a third of our twenty-four-hour day in sleep. For some of that time, we dream. Not everyone remembers their dreams, but sleep studies tell us that we do dream and that sleep and dreaming are vital to our health. Scientists also have found that when we are deprived of sleep and dreaming, our healing, detoxification, mental health, and moods are negatively affected. In sleep and dreams, we plot out solutions to difficulties, plan ahead, practice physical skills, and wake better prepared for the coming day.

My brother has asked me to set down some of my thoughts and experiences in using "dreaming with awareness" for healing. Since it is such a broad topic, I will highlight the following topics to discuss:

- We are dreaming all the time—awake or asleep.

- There are different types of dreams.

- To a certain degree, we can program our sleep and dream experience for our benefit.

- Our bodies and minds are dream catchers that can be put to use. In many traditions, people construct objects called dream catchers. By using certain symbols and invocations, we can tune that dream catcher object to attract the dream experience we want and to filter out the ones we don't. In the same way, we can program our minds and bodies to attract some dream experiences to enrich our lives and, hopefully, filter out those we would rather not encounter.

- There are four gates of lucid dreaming (to be conscious in the dreaming state, or aware that you are dreaming).

- There are certain symbols in dreams that are near universal and others that are personal, many of which can help us gain insight. What is most important is that you get to know your own symbols well so that you can recognize intrusions into your dreams when you encounter them, either from higher guidance or other people.

- The content and texture of our dreams can give us a great deal of information.

- We can receive instruction, training, and advice in our dreams.

- There is a coherence of symbols between daytime and sleep-time dreaming.

- The organ systems and flora have an effect on dreaming. In many traditions, most notably traditional Chinese medicine, each organ system is associated with specific emotions, symbols, colors, and thought patterns. For example, the liver is associated with anger, the kidneys with fear, and the stomach and pancreas with sorrow. (See Chapter 12 for a more complete discussion.) When these systems are out of balance in the body, these emotions will play out in our dreamscape. Since our gut biome is a representation of the microbial environment of our home, land, and dietary habits, different compositions of gut microbiome will affect the background of the dreamscape in different ways. Many of the by-products of indigestion can affect neurotransmitters in the brain and our moods.

Considering that we spend about a third of each day asleep, it is remarkable how little we talk about this aspect of life in the service of healing (beyond the basic need to get "enough sleep"). Here are just a few examples:

- During sleep, the majority of detoxification biochemistry takes place.

- During REM sleep, we practice physical skills thousands of times without the muscle strains and repetitive motion injuries that we could have incurred had we been awake. Sleeping and dreaming is our main recourse for practicing a skill the 10,000 times it takes to make it automatic.

- My first spiritual teacher, Dr. Francisco Coll, taught that during sleep, our "silver cord stretches out to the universe," and we regrouped with the Infinite, hold congress with our angels and other souls, and receive "letters from God."

Certainly, we are all aware that poor and insufficient sleep results in many health and disease challenges, but while we pay a great deal of lip service to the idea of "sleep hygiene," we seem to lack the sophistication to help people who are suffering from insomnia and other sleep difficulties. CPAP machines and melatonin just haven't been the panacea that we prayed for. There is much to do and explore to help folks in this area. I maintain that there are many aspects of sleep time, and the dreaming landscape that accompanies it, that are fertile avenues for a healer to pursue.

In most cultures historically, and even still, a day begins not when the alarm clock prods you to begin your workday, but the evening before. On awakening, we are given a taste of the day in store for us and therefore prepared by Spirit.

THE LANGUAGE AND SYMBOLS OF DREAMS

Dreams use our power of imagination. "Imagination," in its broadest sense, includes all of our sensory faculties, memory, reason, and speech to present us with an experience that feels like reality to us while we are in the midst of a dream. Some have likened dreaming to a theater with only one person in the audience. While dreaming, we see and interact with people, beings, objects, and events. Words are spoken, emotions are felt, and sometimes even background music is playing. Many of us call this dream content the "language" of dreaming because it seems to represent messages from our subconscious and superconscious to our conscious mind. These experiences often give direction, information, and meaning that can be useful for carrying out our life's work with integrity, love, and success.

Some symbols and feelings are derived from input from the physical body, energy body, emotional body, and/or mental body. As such, they can be of great interest to healers. For example, as noted previously, in Chinese medicine each organ system is associated with different emotions—the liver with anger, the lungs with grief and injustice, the kidneys with fear, the heart with excessive joy, the stomach with worry, and the pericardium with frustration and impatience. When these emotions appear in a dream, one might wonder about imbalances in the related organ systems. Also, while pain is absent during unconscious dreamless sleep, pain can be present in sleeping dreams. This pain can correlate with waking pain. Pain that doesn't go away at night raises the specter of organ illness more so than pain that disappears at night.

Dream language is symbolic, poetic, and meaningful. It is often subtle but sometimes direct. In looking at dreams, we are forced to think like spirit does, to see the symbols, conversations, people, manner of dress, and events as poetic, representative, and written in "spirit's" language, which may allow us to grow in our awareness. While dreaming, and then upon awakening from that dream, we have to do our homework, to explore the inner map of our symbols, memories, and feelings. It is an invitation to explore the inner depths of who we are.

The general mood of a dream is also significant. Was it pleasant, fearful, upsetting, frustrating, etc.? This is a good way to begin an inquiry into the possible emotional underpinnings of illness and disease.

Some symbols seem nearly universal: female for feelings, male for intellect, buildings for structure, wallets and credit cards for personal identity and possessions, water for emotions and spirit, prison bars and shackles for feeling constrained, and release from prison or flying for freedom and liberation.

Other symbols are intensely personal. A student of mine saw many images of owls in her dreams. Not surprisingly, owls appeared in person on her walks in nature as well, serving as a sort of confirmation of the message. Each person has a repertoire, or collection, of symbols that appear frequently in their remembered dreams, which signal to them that they are on familiar ground, close to home. This usual "dream space" is their personal dream. When you wander into another dream space, you can recognize it by foreign symbols and feelings, a different texture and landscape to the dream.

Just as you can learn to read what your conscious is trying to communicate through the content and feelings of your dreams, I have found that you can teach your subconscious a symbology that allows you to ask questions, work in your dreams, and heal yourself and others by programming your sleep experience at night and during meditation. This sharpens communication. You can decide that a rose means yes and an anvil means no. Some other symbol or word stands in for your profession, your purpose and thrust. And with repetition, it will start to appear in the nighttime dream space. These same symbols will appear in the midst of your mundane workaday life, allowing a deeper, more intimate, and real-time relationship between you and your integrity. You will feel more and more like Noah, "walking with God." When something is unclear, you can ask for elaboration. You can program yourself to redream the dream, even in a twenty-minute nap.

Not every dream experience is important or significant. What helps us to know which dreams are important is the dream texture. This is a harder concept to describe than to appreciate. There is a normal feel to the ordinary discharge dream—the type of dream that discharges leftover emotions, energies, conflicts, and ideas of the day. It is a mishmash of images, discussion, emotional reactions, movements, and so on. For most people, the mood, content, and imagery in this type of dream are not so different from day-to-day life, chiefly because most of the undigested events, emotions, and information don't really vary that much in the average person's life from day to day. A lot of these "mundane" dreams are simply discharges of leftover feelings and ideas from the daytime. They come out in a rush like a hodgepodge of people coming out of a movie theater.

A mundane dream is a discharge dream. All of the other dreams that I mentioned are important in that they convey specific messages, information, and empowerments to the dreamer. The typical discharge dream doesn't have the focus or the power to do this.

Feeling the texture of a dream is very much an inner knowing. When I ask my patients if the texture of a significant dream was different, they always say "yes." We never need to analyze and dissect why; thus, I call it a "knowing," which is a gift of perception that is addressed in Chapter 2.

THE TEACHINGS OF DON MIGUEL RUIZ

One of the teachers who helped me with dreaming was don Miguel Ruiz, author of the books *The Four Agreements* and *The Mastery of Love.*

Don Miguel is a master of lucid dreaming, and I found, when studying with him, that he would often appear in my nighttime dreams to give me instructions, pointers, and healings. When he appeared in one of my dreams, the entire texture of the dream would shift. Colors were much more vibrant, the sensation in my nerves was incredibly vivid, words rang out with the clarity of a theatrical production, and the dream had an incredibly strong and long-lasting impact afterward. People in this type of dream tend to look like they do in "real life," including the secondary characters. These dreams were memorable to the last detail. I would often awaken immediately at their conclusion, and for days I would return to the memory of the dream, almost magnetically, to sift through them so that I could decipher every drop of teaching.

According to don Miguel, there are four "gates" of significant dreaming:

- The first gate is to wake up in your dream. This is the birth of awareness.

  Don Miguel would work with patients to see if they could awaken in their dream, converse and consciously interact with him, and even take conscious action while still dreaming.

  What do I mean by this? In our dreams, we respond to events and take action. Most of the time, it is only when we awaken that we realize we were dreaming. The "me" who speaks in such a dream is not under the control of the witness who is watching the dream. We say that such a "me" is not awakened in the dream. If this is your dream experience, you have not passed through the first gate.

  Once through the first gate, you can say while you are in the middle of the dream, "Oh, I'm dreaming, how cool." Most of the time, this insight will rouse you immediately. You may notice that the body you inhabit during a dream (referred to as your "dream body") doesn't have much definition in the lower limbs, but this is not universal. You will also discover that if you spend too much time bringing your attention to one object or another in the dream, it will fade away and dissolve, and you will awaken.

- The second gate is to consciously transform the dream you are in. So, you can say, "I am dreaming now. I don't want this dream; let's change it." Then you can move to a new scene or change your conversation to be lighter, healthier, or more satisfying.

- The third gate is being capable of transforming an awakened dream to notice that you are experiencing someone else's dream. In other words, to recognize while still dreaming that the symbols, moods, and textures of a particular sleeping dream don't match the symbols, moods, and textures of your natural dreams. You realize that you are acting as a secondary character in another person's nighttime dream! As a participant in someone else's process, once you have mastered transformation, you can exit that dream if it is not something you want to experience, or you can observe with curiosity what the dream is all about. You have free will.

  I know that this sounds bizarre, but I have to say, having worked with a number of masters, this scenario is very real and very important, as I will describe a bit later. It reflects the fluidity of our dream bodies and our interactions in the dream world.

- The final or fourth gate is where you awaken in someone else's dream and have the ability to transform that dream through your interaction. In other words, you can consciously converse or act in someone else's dream as if you were awake working with others.

Why is any of this relevant, except as entertainment or a demonstration of spiritual power? It is vital to understand that, awake or asleep, we are dreaming all the time.

Don Miguel taught that it is far more important to wake up in your daily life (which we think of as the "real world") than to do so in your nighttime sleeping dreams. Our waking experience of life has much in common with the nighttime sleep world. Don Miguel taught during Toltec Dreaming that the chief difference between daytime and nighttime dreaming is that the "frame" of a daytime dream is constant, whereas the frame of a sleeping dream is in constant flux.

What is true of a waking dream is that houses are houses, desks are desks, and gravity works as it typically does. You don't blink your eyes and find that the city you live in has transformed itself into Rome, or Antarctica, or outer space. This is what we mean when we refer to the "frame of the dream."

Like the dream at night, in the daytime, we are constantly moving from one thought to another, one scene to another, one mood and sensation to another. Certain images and words stick out to us in both dreams, while others seem evanescent and indistinct. Many of our actions while awake are automatic, reflexive, and not thought through with clarity, just like observing ourselves in the nighttime dream as if we were watching a movie, that sort of concerns us but isn't vivid, alive, or under our conscious control. Most of us can't really extract ourselves from an unpleasant situation in a moment, or change the outcome of a daytime dream, except here and there. We move through the waking dream—the real world—semiconscious, aware of some of the people we meet and oblivious of others, sometimes noticing the scenery around us and at other times living entirely in our own fantasies.

Perhaps the most curious thing about our daytime dream is the subjective experience of living. Each of us might have gone to the same nightclub or movie or participated in the same conversation, but no two people experience a real-life event in the exact same way. It really is a dream!

How many times do we have a moment of insight, realizing that the meal we just ate, the night we spent in front of the computer, or even our entire relationship with someone was essentially experienced unconscious and asleep. In that moment, we have crossed the first gate of dreaming in our waking life: we have begun to wake up.

Even when we are sleepwalking through life—through our daily routines, our jobs, our marriages—the events that happen to us have impact. While asleep, we can overeat, forget personal hygiene, be unconsciously cruel to ourselves and others, and fail to be present with our loved ones. This is the price we pay for being asleep while thinking we are awake.

Many of my patients have had adverse childhood experiences (ACEs), defined as traumatic experiences before the age of eighteen that contribute to morbidity and mortality. ACEs happen when an entire family is essentially asleep, responding reflexively to each other's words and gestures, not realizing what they are doing.

Can we wake up in real life and know that we are dreaming, stop automatic responses, and create a new reality for ourselves? Can we understand when we are in the grip of someone else's dream, whether it is our boss, our spouse, our parents, or our child? And can we do something about it to effect a positive outcome?

Practice in the nighttime dream is the playground for transforming our daytime lives. And just as certain daytime experiences stand out as more consequential than others, most people will agree that there are different categories of nighttime dreams.

TYPES OF NIGHTTIME DREAMS

The most common dream for most people is the discharge dream, in which undigested events, information, interactions, and emotions from the daytime are carried over to the night, processed, digested, and discharged. In a discharge dream, we have a window into this process. Fears and frustrations, information, and impactful images all coalesce into a mishmash of experiences that never quite rise to a coherent whole. We are left with some intriguing clues to our inner process, but not the entire picture.

The second category of dream is the powerful dream. This type of dream leaves us with a definite impression that something important happened or was conveyed to us. Many times, they are teaching or healing dreams. (The dreams with don Miguel Ruiz that I experience fit within this category.) The texture and impact are different. We tend to remember them longer, and if we write them down, they often have meaning long into the future. Even if we cannot completely understand them at the time, we know that something happened to us. Over the years, nearly all of my students have reported to me that at one time or another I appeared in their dreams and gave them specific and powerful teachings.

The third category of dream is the dream of power. A dream of power is another textual dream, full of vibrancy and impact. What distinguishes it from other types is that in this dream, you take an action that transcends your previous state of consciousness, carrying you to a higher level of awareness and agency in your life. For example, perhaps you have been having recurring dreams about someone attacking you, putting you down, or confining you. One day, in a dream, you respond differently: you get up, break free, or fight back. Upon awakening, you are likely to feel a sense of exhilaration or freedom, a lightening. That is a dream of power. When this watershed event happens, the energy of your entire approach to life shifts as well. You recover a big piece of your personal power.

Prophetic dreams are rare events for most people. Still, most people will have at least one in their lifetime. In this type of dream, you see the future clearly, or you witness present events that are taking place in a distant location not normally known to you. They are not always pleasant events, either. In the dream state, I have seen the passing of a friend's son from leukemia, the loss of a lawsuit for another friend, and the unexpected breakup of a relationship. In the dream about my friend's son's death, I saw the baby appear in front of me and then shrink into the distance bit by bit. The next moment the phone rang, and I received the news. In all of these cases, the texture of the dream was not usual.

Finally, we should discuss lucid dreams. Different experts give varying definitions of what a lucid dream is. Some people who claim expertise in dreaming call vivid, outstanding dreams about colorful adventures lucid. Other experts require that the individual be awake in the dream and control the direction and dialogue of their own role. There is an elaborate and extended narrative about training to do so and what can be done with lucid dreaming in the shamanic traditions. Carlos Castaneda's books, such as *The Art of Dreaming,* are good textbooks for those who wish to practice and develop this art.

A waking lucid dream is often called a *vision.*

EMPTYING AND SETTING THE STAGE

If you want to increase your percentage of lucid dreams of power, you need to prepare the environment of your nighttime activity. I will share with you a technique that I use with many of my patients who are suffering from insomnia due to a racing mind.

I call this technique "emptying and setting the stage." The idea behind emptying is that if you have not fully digested the day's events, interactions, ideas, and projects, you have to use nighttime dreaming to finish the job. Thus, your dreams will likely be discharge dreams, detoxifying the remains of the day rather than inspiring you to a healthy future. In emptying, you sit for a few minutes and review the day as if watching a movie. As you review each episode, you exhale the residue of emotions, energy, and so on as you turn your head slowly from side to side. As you practice this, the events of your day will appear to you, often in chronological order. Certain interactions or experiences will stand out, while others will be brought to mind that you have forgotten completely. People who were in the background, but who shared with you some significant exchange, will come to mind. All of this will show you how rich your life is and relieve a lot of pressure, tension, and stress. Some interactions will not clear easily, even with breathing. Put them on a shelf and wish them well. With time, they will lose their intensity.

The next step is setting the stage. Using your imagination, envision the day ahead as a road or trail. First, look and see how it is: is it smooth, straight, split, winding, rough, or full of obstacles? Next, take an imaginary brush or broom and sweep the path clear, straighten it out, and make it even. Now, take an imaginary paint can and brush the day ahead with the mood of your choice: relaxation, ease, love, surprise, adventure, camaraderie, and so on. Imagine placing boxes of energy with your mind's eye all along the route that you can tap into whenever your energy flags. Next, put signposts along the way so that you can be directed back to your plan whenever your get lost or stray; add companions or friends; include depots of resources, such as money and time; and let your way be dusted by angels or friendly beings to give support, guidance, and boosting as needed. Finally, ask your inner guidance any questions you would like answered in the night and thank the universe for another day, hoping that all beings are happy in all worlds.

Simple? Yes. Yet incredibly effective.

To get traction with this exercise or any other will take practice, which just means repetition.

PRACTICAL USES OF DREAMING

For me, the chief use of dreaming is in learning new techniques and approaches to healing. Sometime, this is in response to an earnest inquiry that I have made. I often pose a question to myself and my inner guidance before I hit the pillow at night. The answer might come in a dream or, very often, in the first few minutes of waking, perhaps while I am in the shower or brushing my teeth. It comes to me as a "knowing," a direct insight with great clarity that feels complete and settled when I direct my attention to the impression.

One of the most valuable insights came to me one morning in the shower. I had been perplexed, wondering why on some days I awoke refreshed and calm, and other days I would awaken with aches, pains, moodiness, and sometimes obsessions, particularly over financial issues. I took this question to bed. In the morning, I had a "tape" running through my brain about something I believed I had put to bed years ago. It was an obsessive thought. As usual, I began an internal conversation that went, "Here we go again!" At that moment, an insight that was a knowing came to me: "Are you sure this belongs to you? Maybe you are feeling the world or the people around you?" What was really remarkable about this insight was that the instant it came to me, the obsessive voices in my head stopped—completely! As a conscientious self-help practitioner, I had come to believe, as many do, that my moods and ideas are my own, and they result from my thinking and are subject to my intentional efforts. The idea that some of what comes to me is not mine immediately felt suspicious, as if I was dodging my responsibilities and putting them on others.

For me, three questions followed:

- If this mood, feeling, or obsessive thought isn't coming from me, where is it coming from and what does it mean? Could it be my inner sensitivity picking up on the mood of the community in general, or even one or more of my patients or colleagues I am to encounter this very day?

- If the latter is true, can I make use of it as a diagnostic tool that can help me understand the behavior of people around me, and possibly even some of the underpinnings of disease in my patients?

- How can I test to see whether it is me or not?

For many months, I observed carefully my morning moods, dream moods, and penetrating thoughts and obsessions in addition to my clientele, colleagues, and community. Sure enough, it seemed that when I questioned whether a given thought or feeling was mine, it disappeared. There was a strong correlation with the most challenging patients on my schedule for the day, or colleagues, or anyone I encountered in my daily life who would tell me about their moods, insecurities, and obsessions. There was a one-to-one correlation with the morning feelings and the world of the day!

I also realized that if the unpleasant mood, thought, or sensation went away immediately after I asked whether it was mine, then it definitely was not mine. Most of the time it was not hard to figure out where it had come from—a disgruntled colleague, a worrying partner or child, or a patient I was to meet for the first time. But if the situation persisted after I asked the key question, it meant that it did belong to me; it came from my mind, and I had to clear it up in my personal processing.

Once I became comfortable with this technique, I began to refine it: I developed a self-inquiry, which I call "spheres of influence," that allows me to pinpoint more directly the source of the impression. These spheres include my home environment, my work environment, my colleagues, my patients, my friends and family, and lastly, the community at large.

So, if I began my morning by thinking about how assets grew with compounding interest and what it would take to reach a certain financial goal (a topic I was not really interested in otherwise), I would check that sphere of influence: if it were colleagues, I would gently inquire of my coworkers how things were going in the marketplace. Invariably, what would follow would be a lecture on Wall Street and a description of their ambitions, their financial plans, and, of course, their worries.

If it the thought was coming from a patient, I could inquire, "Are there any issues with money in the family?" Invariably, I would hear, after a sigh, "Things are challenging at the moment." Or the patient would explain the events of a reversal of fortune that immediately preceded their chronic complaint.

Another boon from this process was that I would often awaken with a deep insight about a clinical situation that had confused me—a line of treatment or diagnosis—and that would much more often than not prove to be the linchpin of clinical success for the patient. Along with these clinical "pearls," at times the insight would be so significant that it opened up an entirely new treatment tool, an avenue for research, or an approach to a broad band of patients with particular problems.

For example, in trying to figure out how to care for certain patients with refractory SIBO (small intestinal bacterial overgrowth), I awoke with the idea and a mental picture of combining "impacho" massage, which is a massage of the intestinal tract for moving stagnation along, with Bach flower remedies and German biologicals applied topically over the various abdominal organs, touched up with electrical acupuncture stimulation of low-resistance places on the abdominal wall. I have since found this combination to be incredibly useful for resolving digestive issues in many people.

Let me also recount a recent experience that I had with a patient regarding dreams at night. Florence called me to say that she'd had a really interesting dream and asked for my reflection. In this dream, she found three credit cards in her hand that she didn't realize she owned. She thought they belonged to her parents (who in real life had passed away a number of years ago). She knew that it was important for her to return these cards to her parents and asked herself how to find them. A staircase appeared at once but didn't feel right to her. A second staircase appeared, and when she ascended those stairs, she met her father and mother. The reunion was incredibly emotional for her, and she wept inside the dream. She returned the cards and woke up.

My first question was about the texture of the dream. Was it unusual? Yes! I asked her if there was something she felt she owed her parents. Of course, a flood of emotion came. She said that she had hoped to tell them how much she loved and appreciated them while they were alive but had procrastinated and didn't get to do it. In fact, she had donated money to her parents' alma mater, where they had met. To me, that effort felt like the first staircase; Florence agreed.

So perhaps the second staircase was a new way of working. I felt moved to share with her a variety of techniques to clear unresolved conflicts, traumas, and wounds from her matrilineal and patrilineal histories and to create a gratitude ritual. This immediately led to a lifting of mood and a great healing. I don't yet know if this realization translated into relief of some of the physical symptoms that had come on for Florence since the death of her parents, but I would not be surprised if it did.

I hope this chapter has given you a good overview of some of the rewards of dreaming work in the life of a healer that can help the people they work with.

Gene Nathan, MD, is a board-certified pediatrician, integrative physician, and spiritual teacher. At a young age, he found healing and medicine to be his calling. After medical school, he became a board certified pediatrician, studied homeopathy with Robin Murphy, trained in clinical acupuncture, energy healing with Dr. Francisco Coll, studied tai chi and chi gong at the Taoist Sanctuary of San Diego and Toltec Dreaming with don Miguel Ruiz, MD, for eight years, and collaborated with Dr. Vijith (Ayurvedic practitioner) in India. His interest in children, families, and societal health led him to a fellowship in infant mental health, where he studied with Dr. Brazelton and others. He has worked to set up community programs in child development in San Diego that have helped many thousands of families through the American Academy of Pediatrics. He currently practices in Driggs, Idaho, working with concussions, complex illnesses, autoimmune conditions, and other brain disorders, bringing a multimodal approach to help those who have not received the help they need from Western medicine. Contact him through drgeneintegrativemed. com, or reach him at genenathanconsults@gmail.com.

PART III
Other Important Energetic Considerations: Expanding Our Awareness

It was always my intention to include a section in this book on how we obtain information from nature. We humans are mammals, of course, and always have been members of the natural world. But, as we evolved, we somehow decided that we were the pinnacle of evolution and had progressed to the point that our knowledge permitted us to determine what was best for all living creatures. Yes, we were aware that there were other sentient beings around us, such as dolphins, whales, and other primates, but we slowly came to believe that our needs outweighed other considerations.

When humans emerged on this planet, they were an integral part of that world, and virtually all "primitive" cultures operated out of an appreciation for the bounty of food and other resources that were available to them for survival. They lived in harmony with nature, and it was important that balance was maintained. Ever so slowly as to be almost imperceptible, humankind lost sight of that balance and its place within it.

Fast-forward to the twenty-first century. It appears to me that our fascination with technology is moving into a higher gear. We seem to be embracing the development of artificial intelligence (AI) as our future. Science fiction writers, often the visionaries of what may be possible someday, have warned us about this outcome for decades. A goal toward which we may be heading—the next step of our evolution—is the use of neural implants directly into the brain that would allow people to access vast amounts of data and process it at lightning-fast speeds.

This scenario is probably closer to reality than I care to admit, because it terrifies me. While the idea that we will be able to process information at unheard-of rates is intriguing, it also seems clear to me that this focus on cold, hard data is already distancing us from what makes us human—our connection to the natural world and all that is alive in it. We have begun to define ourselves by the numbers of "hits" we notice when we are Googled, or by the number of "friends" we have on Facebook, or how many "likes" we get rather than by the meaningful conversations we have with our neighbors.

Perhaps I am a dinosaur, and all of this progress will enable us to move into an ideal future, but so far I see little evidence of this. I do not see how this focus on technology has enabled us to appreciate the planet we inhabit and take care of it as if it was truly our home. In writing this book, an important part of the message I was hoping to send was to remind us of our connection to plants and all other beings on this Earth and help us realize that these connections are central to our future.

It is no secret that in clear-cutting forests, developing and releasing tens of thousands of untested chemicals into the environment, and exposing ourselves to unprecedented amounts of electromagnetic energies, we have produced a toxic planet that humans are genetically unequipped to deal with. As I noted before but believe is worth repeating, the current epidemics of cancer, autism, autoimmune disease, chronic fatigue syndrome, fibromyalgia, neurodegenerative disease, Lyme disease, and mold toxicity are harbingers of what our lack of caring for our own Earth is creating. As I write these words, we are in the midst of the COVID-19 pandemic, and scientists tell us that there are more deadly outbreaks to come.

As I wrote this part of the book, it evolved into an effort to point out that human history has, until recently, always included an appreciation of the natural world and humanity's place in it. In Chapter 15, I will discuss communication with plants. Chapter 16 delves into the relationship between native healers and the natural world and what it can teach us about this important subject.

I believe there is a desperate need for us to be reminded about embracing our heritage so that we can get back into balance with ourselves and all of the sentient beings who share this world.

CHAPTER 15:
Communicating with Plants and Other Life Forms

How to See the Forest AND the Trees

There are numerous reports that plants respond well to certain stimuli. Many folks who are blessed with "green thumbs" attribute the health and growth of their plants to being talked to, being sung to, or having music played for them. Yes, these claims are easy to dismiss, but they are made so often that it might be reasonable to take them seriously.

My own eyes were opened to this possibility in the spring of 1982 when I attended the annual conference of the American Holistic Medical Association in Chicago with several colleagues. There were three of us: myself; my dear friend Carolyn Torkelson, who at the time worked with me as a nurse practitioner (she later became a physician and still teaches at the University of Minnesota); and another nurse practitioner named Patricia. Having little money at that time, we drove home from the meeting together. Realizing that we would not be able to get back to Minnesota at a reasonable hour, we decided to camp overnight in the Black River State Forest in southern Wisconsin. The weather was balmy and we had sleeping bags with us, so we were disappointed to find that the park had not yet opened for the season. We decided to park outside the gate and walk in with our gear anyway. To our delight, we found a simple gazebo with a sandy floor, climbed into our bags, and fell asleep.

The next morning, we each arose at our own time and went to explore the park independently. I wandered off on one of the paths and felt compelled to walk up a short rise. At the top, I had the oddest sensation. A plant there seemed to want to communicate with me.

I do not have the words to explain how, but after I sat down on the trail in front of the plant, it clearly explained to me that it was a "wisdom" plant and that if its leaves were prepared in a certain way, the person who consumed them would gain some degree of insight in a particular area. It was also clear to me that I was not to pick the plant, but simply to learn about this possibility. I was left with the amazing feeling that this plant had literally sought me out and explained to me its use for humans.

After a while, I wandered back to join my companions. To our mutual surprise, both of my friends had had very similar experiences. As we shared the events of the morning, we discovered that each of us had been led to a different section of the park and "told" about the use of a particular plant for healing. We were dumbfounded by our extraordinary experience. None of us had any inkling that this sort of communication was possible, yet we all were clear that it had indeed occurred. While I never identified this plant, that was not the point of this experience…it was only to show me, at a profound level, that plants can, and do, communicate to us directly if we are open to that possibility.

For me, this experience clarified a mystery that I had pondered for some time. How did "primitive" cultures learn about the use of plants? It was hard to imagine that purely trial-and-error experiments eventually led to the knowledge of how to use plants for healing and nurturance. Our forebears would have had so many negative reactions to plant toxins involving nausea, vomiting, palpitations, diarrhea, muscle twitching and cramps, and even death to discourage the wanton experimentation that would have been required to obtain this information. My companions and I came to the realization that gaining this knowledge did not require risking life and limb; the plants "told" us how to use them properly, and we "listened." As far-fetched as it may seem, the quality and intensity of this experience left me no doubt that communicating with plants was not only possible but was a reality.

STEPHEN HARROD BUHNER AND THE LOST LANGUAGE OF PLANTS

Many years later, I read the remarkable books by Stephen Harrod Buhner, the eminent herbalist, philosopher, and poet, whose vivid descriptions of how we communicate with and learn from plants validated our experience in the park. I had hoped that he would be able to write this next section himself. Since that was not possible, he provided me with the next best option, giving me permission to quote from his many books to help us understand these vital concepts.

Buhner is probably best known for his groundbreaking books on a variety of infectious illnesses and their herbal treatments. What makes these books unique is that they are written from the point of view of the microbe. Rather than accept the current medical model that these infectious agents are "bad" and need to be eradicated by the strongest antibiotic available, Buhner comes to the table with a different approach, asking important questions such as

- What do these microbes need from us?

- What is the nature of this interaction?

- How do the microbes meet those needs?

- How can we utilize this information to create a healthier treatment approach that is more in sync with the natural order of things?

Let's use the bacterial infection of *Bartonella* (a common coinfection of Lyme disease) as an example. In his 2013 book *Healing Lyme Disease Coinfections,* Buhner helps us understand that this bacteria does not want to kill us, but simply wants to use us as a host. Its first priority is to create ongoing inflammation in our bodies that serves as a major distraction to our immune system, which gets so busy putting out fires that it doesn't quite get around to dealing with the infection that is causing them. Another feature of *Bartonella* is that, like all bacteria, it finds certain human tissues more conducive to its needs, namely our red blood cells and spleen. Utilizing this information, a treatment program should include strategies for decreasing inflammation and supporting the health of the spleen and red blood cells. Buhner lays out in detail a wide variety of herbal treatments that can do so, along with herbs that specifically kill *Bartonella.* This way, he uses natural materials rather than the synthetic antibiotics to which we subject our ecosystem in massive amounts. His approach to understanding and treating these infections has influenced thousands of physicians to begin to approach treatment differently.

On a related note, on page 116 of *The Lost Language of Plants,* Buhner reminds us:

In 1942 the entire world's supply of chemical antibiotics was 32 liters of penicillin.... By 1999—in the United States alone—this figure had grown to an incredible 50 million pounds a year of scores of antibiotics, most of them now synthetic.... Yearly, American factory farms dispense 20 million pounds of antibiotics so food animals will survive overcrowding and fatten for market.

Bacteria have been on this planet billions of years longer than humans have. As astonishing as this concept may seem, they have demonstrated a remarkable capacity to interact with their environment and, as we will see, literally create life as we know it. In the face of this massive threat of antibiotic exposure, bacteria have not been passive. Their innate abilities allow them to develop resistance to these antibiotics and then share that information with their bacterial colleagues (a phenomenon well documented in medicine); in other words, the bacteria not only survive the threat but become resistant to it. You likely have read about "superbugs," which are no longer susceptible to our antibiotics due to overuse. Many medical experts fear that antibiotics will be unable to treat many common infections in the near future. An excellent example of this is MRSA, a penicillin-resistant staph infection. It has become a serious problem in hospitals; many patients come in for a minor procedure and leave with a life-threatening infection that does not respond to antibiotic treatment.

Let's try to put into context what this means to humans, plants, and all life forms on Earth. On page 57, Buhner says:

[Evolutionary biologist] Lynn Margulis discovered that all complex life developed from an original symbiosis of four different bacteria: *archaebacteria*, *spirochetes*, *cyanobacteria*, and oxygen-breathing bacteria. After this early unification, other kinds of bacteria were incorporated into the structures of cells.

Medical science has confirmed that the mitochondria, the crucial organelles in our cells that provide us with both energy and protection, have their own DNA, which is identical to that of bacteria. This clearly shows that we have a millennia-long relationship with bacteria and rely on them for our very existence. Each of us has approximately 70 trillion bacteria living in our intestinal tract that are essential to our well-being and form the complex ecosystem of our gut, which we rely on for so many physiological needs.

So, if we contemplate that massive amount of synthetic antibiotics released into our environment along with radioactive waste (including a great deal of medical waste), the 80,000 chemicals to which we are exposed in the form of cleaning products, food additives, and manufactured products (the vast majority of which have not been tested on humans or any other life form), and the presence of unimaginable electromagnetic wave exposure that has never before been known in human existence, we have to ask ourselves, what are we doing?

Plants, too, have bacterial ancestry. As Buhner notes on page 58:

> Bacteria are, in essence, the primary life form on Earth.... Chloroplasts—originally cyanobacteria—were incorporated into the majority of plant cells on Earth. It is the chloroplasts that make plants green, engage in photosynthesis, and turn power from the sun into the food and energy that enables plants to live.

The bottom line here is that, in our hubris, we are interfering with the natural order without understanding the consequences. With the best of intentions (thinking we could stamp out infectious illness as our love affair with antibiotics began), we have created a global threat.

If you can embrace what has been discussed thus far, it is not a big leap to understand the Gaia hypothesis as proposed by British chemist James Lovelock in the 1960s and co-developed by Lynn Margulis in the 1970s. Gaia, "the ancient Greek name for the living, intelligent, and sacred Earth," was suggested by the novelist William Golding. Buhner writes on page 172, "This recognition of Earth's self-regulating nature led Lovelock to understand Earth as a living being, not a ball of resources inhabited by human beings hurtling through space." Within this understanding:

> Each plant, plant neighborhood, ecosystem, and biome has messages flowing through it constantly—trillions and trillions of messages at the same time. The messages are complex communications between all the different parts of the ecosystem.... Life is so closely coupled with the physical and chemical environment of which it is a part that the two cannot legitimately viewed in isolation from one another.

This is the bigger picture. If it seems like a bit much to take in all at once, let's come back to plants, the primary subject of this chapter (but everything is interrelated). With the basic premise that plants have inhabited this planet for much longer than we have, Buhner reminds us on page 174:

> It is our temporal limitations that prevent most of us from noticing what plants do over scales of time. For instance, from recognizing that plants and plant communities possess tremendous powers of movement, that their movement shows intention, that they can cross thousands of miles when motivated, and that their movement patterns are not random but are determined by large-scale feedback loops millions of years old.... Plants circulate throughout ecosystems, between ecosystems and across and

between continents; the longest seed dispersal distance known (without human help) is 15,000 miles. Plants, in fact, move themselves throughout landmasses and across distances that mere seed dispersal dynamics and mathematics cannot explain. The places they move to and the ways that they arrange themselves in ecosystems are not accidental and are not random.... they arrange themselves to fulfill specific functions; their spatial arrangements exist for a reason.

Buhner provides many examples. On page 183 he says:

Elder trees...are keystone species in many ecosystems. Among many indigenous and folk peoples it is said that the Elder tree 'teaches the plants what to do and how to grow' and that without its presence the local plant community will become confused.... Keystone species regulate the broad community dynamics of a plant community (its character), while the smaller community species regulate the flow of life to and through it: pollinators, "critical pests, pathogens, herbivores or mutualists."

This communication is largely done through chemical mediators made by the plants. On page 146, Buhner lists 130 different chemicals known to be present in a single yarrow plant. Just as we humans utilize neurotransmitters to send information, plants can make and distribute different chemicals to different areas to orchestrate their environment. Through their roots, leaves, flowers, pollens, saps, and other secretions, they communicate with each other and with other plant, insect, and animal species (including humans if we would just listen). Buhner provides numerous examples of how plants then influence the insect and animal species that share their environment to create the complexity of life in that ecosystem.

Buhner goes on to say on page 197 that

deeper awareness of the sophisticated complexity of plant chemistries and the inextricably interwoven connection of plants and their chemistries to the life around them has begun to reveal to contemporary peoples that plant chemistries are used not only for the plants themselves, but are created and released to heal disease throughout the ecosystems in which they grow. For example, in plant communities, the closely intertwined feedback loops automatically note when any member of the plant community is ill and the mycelial networks just under the surface of the soil transport necessary chemistries to it.

He cites many fascinating examples of this, for one noting on page 198 that

> Bee pollinators, most notably honeybees, collect a gummy resinous substance from trees to make propolis, which they use to coat the interior of their hive to protect it from infection.... The bees combine the tree resins with nectars, multiple pollens, wax, and the bees' internal enzymes. Propolis...is strongly antibacterial, antiviral, antibiotic, antifungal, anti-inflammatory antioxidant and antiseptic.... Many of the trees that propolis is collected from, such as willow, birch, aspen and poplar, exude compounds rich in salicylic acid, which contributes to the strong anti-inflammatory properties of propolis.

As another example, he notes, "Many birds collect a variety of fresh, strongly medicinal plants and weave them into their nests to prevent and treat pest infestations or boost the immune activity of their young."

Buhner makes a strong argument that as one studies the natural world and begins to understand it, it becomes increasingly obvious that this world did not evolve by accident. The more details you can delve into (and he provides many such examples), the clearer it is that this is an incredibly complicated, coordinated dance, and all of the players have consciousness and intent in creating this interaction, which goes far beyond words. It cannot be understood by mere mental efforts; it must be felt viscerally.

Perhaps now it does not seem so far-fetched that plants can, and do, communicate with us as well. If only we were not quite so arrogant to assume that other life forms were not sentient and did not have anything to tell us. They do!

By the end of *The Lost Language of Plants,* on page 223 Buhner helps us understand that

> there are holes inside all of us. Holes that can only be filled by certain plants...Emptiness that can only be filled by some of the other life of this Earth. Other life with which we have evolved through a million years of evolution. Without filling them we live a half-life, never becoming fully human, never being healed or whole or completely who we are.

Perhaps this gives us a tiny glimpse into why so many of us are so captivated by our pets or our gardens. We need them at least as much as they need us.

BUHNER AND THE SECRET TEACHINGS OF PLANTS

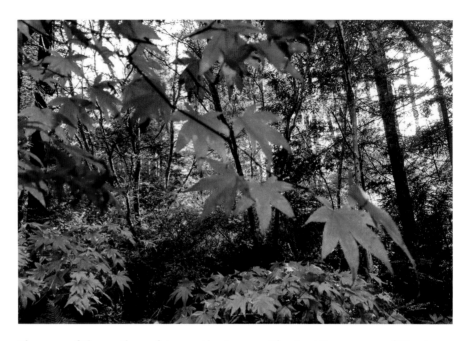

If some of these thoughts captivate you, *The Lost Language of Plants* is only an appetizer. The next book in the series, *The Secret Teachings of Plants,* delves into communication with plants in a more direct and profound way. Buhner has divided the information into two distinct parts. Part One, titled "Systole: Of Nature and the Heart," attempts to explain this communication from a left-brained (analytical) perspective, using intricate information and arguments to make it accessible. Part Two (the one that resonates with me), titled "Diastole: Gathering Knowledge from the Heart of the World," uses a right-brained (creative) approach. Buhner jumps right into this subject with:

> You must ask yourself, in the beginning, if you truly want to communicate with plants, just what is the status of the plant? Just how do you really feel about it? Is that plant, there, the one near to your hand, your equal? If you do not feel that it is at least the same to you as a human being (it is better if you understand it is superior), then I am not sure it will talk to you...the first step in learning to talk to plants is cultivating politeness, realizing that the pine trees that have been here for 700 million years must have been doing something before we came on the scene a mere million years ago besides pining away for our existence.

The next step is to respect your elders...

Sensing the world around us is the next essential step, for the linear mind halts its activity in the face of sensory input from the wildness of the world:

"Sensory input takes the place of internal chatter."

Our senses are meant to perceive the world. They developed with and from the world, not in isolation. Using them is the act that opens the door that is Nature....

Our sensory organs are meant to perceive the world. The sensory capacities of human ears were shaped by sounds of the world, our smell formed through long association with the delicate chemistries of plants, our touch by the nonlinear, multidimensional surfaces of Earth, our sight from immersion within the world. They are part of Earth, an expression of communicative contact subtly refined and shaped through long association...

So allow yourself to sense once again. Allow your sensory perception to be your thinking. Sense instead of think...

it's time to come to your senses

Perceiving through the senses opens the door...

Thus, the second act of courage is deciding to trust your senses...to use them as they are meant to be used, as a channel to the world in which you were born.... And to use your senses most productively, you must go out from the cities...you must find a place where Nature is not buried under concrete and asphalt.... To begin to cultivate depth perception of Nature, to gather knowledge directly from plants, go to the plants themselves. Take a walk someplace wild, where the civilized do not go....

Take a few deep breaths when you arrive, settling yourself down deep in your body. Then begin to walk. And as you walk, become sensitive to the feel of Earth under your feet. Notice how it forces your body to move differently than a sidewalk does.... Different muscles are needed in Nature than those that are used in cities.

Now, let yourself drop down into your feet, your feet becoming sensing organs themselves, supportive organs. Let go of holding yourself up, let your feet hold you. And let the reality of Earth come through their touching into you:

a mother's embrace...

As your body becomes more and more alive through the activation of your senses, sensing is what you do instead of thinking.... Your consciousness begins to move out of the brain, leaving the analytic mind behind. You begin to find the world that our ancient ancestors knew so well.... Always, if you allow yourself to notice, one plant will seem more interesting than all the others. It is to this one that you must go. **"**

Buhner now provides careful instructions about how to interact with this plant, utilizing all of your senses to promote the possibility of direct communication, which will, of course, be nonverbal.

" Using direct perception to learn the medicinal powers of plants is not a spectator sport.... Become aware of the feelings that arise in you as you sit by the plant. How do you feel? Now you are learning to see—not merely the physical form of things but the meanings that each thing expresses....

Plants will, if genuinely asked, respond to you. They will teach you their medicine, as plants have always taught human beings. And though human beings may lose the knowledge of the medicinal uses of a plant, the plant always remembers what its medicine is. And they will tell you....

For the power to heal is in the meaning; its chemical form serves only a secondary function. It contains the meaning but it is not the meaning.... For it is the meaning, the spirit of the plant, that heals the disease. The plant merely gives it a form in which to travel. **"**

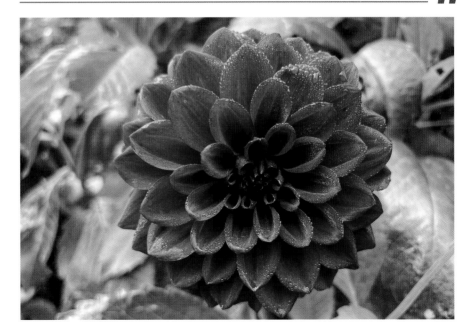

To keep our focus on these ideas and how they can enhance our ability to diagnose and treat patients, Buhner's next chapter, "Depth Diagnosis and the Healing of Human Disease," takes this process and brilliantly translates it into a method for connection with humans, identical to that used with plants, to enable us to understand the disease process in the service of healing.

> This way of gathering knowledge can be used with phenomena other than plants, of course. It can also be used for understanding illness and the healing of disease. The use of direct perception for diagnosis is an extremely elegant way of truly knowing, not thinking, what is going on inside the body.... The process is the same as that used to find the medicinal use of a plant. Only now your gaze is directed at a person. The intention is to know that person's disease, the diseased organ itself, and what it needs....
>
> You are feeling the electromagnetic spectrum of encoded energies, information that the phenomena emits as a specific grouping of feelings. These feelings must be enhanced.... Always asking "What is truly wrong? What is happening to you? Let me see you...." Through this process you enter the territory of disease and healing, weave with it as a participatory consciousness, holding yourself at the fulcrum point, and become the channel through which resolution can occur. There is, in consequence, a deep necessity for you to learn to not fear this territory, to learn to walk within it without letting your fear stop you.... There will sometimes be a tendency, too, when empathy is being established, for your body to entrain with the person's, to take on his disease complex, his physical patterning. You can, if you know your body well enough, allow this to continue until your body itself is (temporarily) ill in just the same manner. Then, by an internal examination of your body, you can see exactly how the disease is manifesting, and what it needs in order to be healed. And, knowing your body so well, you can then allow it to return to its natural functioning....
>
> > *the sufferer is your teacher*
> > *and you must be livingly present*
> > *to learn why*

To illustrate this process in more detail, I wish to quote directly from Buhner's example of how he interacted with a woman who came to him for help. It also gives you a glimpse into the poetic language by which he writes and lives.

"
The woman who had come to see me was tentative at the door, hesitant. Her eyes were nervous, quick, surrounded by lines of worry. She eddied in the door like a wisp of smoke, whispered across the room, and hovered lightly in the chair. She was forty-five years old, short, thin and wiry. Her skin was pale, washed out, her hair a brown, not-flowing shadow of life. Just there.

She had come because she could not breathe. She had asthma.

I said hello as she sat, began drinking tea, telling me her life in many languages. In words. In the small flutterings of her hands. In intonations, the rise and fall of her voice as she spoke. In the slight shifts of her body, in the tiny patterns of emotion that crossed her face. The shape of her body. The clothes she wore.

Her asthma had come on suddenly with no prior history. It had been almost twenty years now. Her medications were many, expensive. Laden with side effects.

I responded to her gesturings of communication. Talked with part of my mind

hearing her speak of her life

while another part looked deeper, seeking the path the disease had taken in her. Searching for traces of its truth.

Her chest caught my attention, standing forth of its own accord, beckoning.

My attention centered there and I breathed into it, letting my awareness move deeper, touching its shape. Feeling my way. I felt a sadness come over me, an overwhelming urge to cry. And then my chest began to feel tight. The muscles clenched, closed down. I began to hunch over slightly, curl around myself. My chest hollowed and I began to breathe high up, rapidly, in small quick bursts of breathing. My breathing a tiny bird, fluttering against the walls of my chest.

I began to feel afraid, slightly hysterical.

I calmed myself, breathed more deeply. Sat back in my chair. Felt a wave of relaxation flow through my muscles. Slowly, one by one, they unclenched.

I let myself care for her then. Sent out a wave of caring from me, to her. Let it touch her chest, hold it in the hollow of caring hands. Waited...waited...waited. Breathing slowly, softly, calmly. Into her chest. Slightly urging it, slowly…slowly…slowly, to relax, to calm down, to breathe… **"**

As Buhner established a connection with this woman, and as she began to open up to him and became less protective of herself, he was able to go deeper into this process:

" I turned my attention back again to her lungs. Letting myself sink deep within in, I began to look.

There was a slight hesitation, like pushing against a mushy blanket, soft cotton wool. A resistance. I sent my caring into the resistance and deeper through it, into her lungs. Asked them to let me see. I stayed present, breathed into the experience. I enhanced the strength of my caring. Looked deeper, focused my seeing, wanted to see.

There was a slight hesitation again. Then a sudden movement into a still, quiet center. And I could see, could feel, the living reality of her lungs.

Their color was off. Some strange cross between gray and mucusy-white. It was old mucus, an unhealthy brownish-yellow glue. My nose wrinkled slightly as the smell came to me…a sick smell, my stomach nauseous to its touch.… Hers [mucus] was dead, unmoving, held in place. Old and unattended. Its life force was gone.… the lungs were slowed down in their function, held back by this oldness.…

Then I felt the need of her lungs and let it flow through me and out, attaching it to my prayer for help so that they flowed together, interweaving with one another, flowing as one earnest need and plea.

I felt that living communication flowing out, its field spreading wide, touching the living reality of the world.… A deep caring and loving came back from the wildness of the world. The world from which all of us have come.

> *And into my mind flashed an image of skunk cabbage*
>
> *powerful, green,*
>
> *luminescent in wetland forest.*

I relaxed my touch then; my concentration softened. My focused awareness let go. And still talking with her with that other part of my mind, I came back into the room, and let these new understandings flow into my talking. I began to weave the healing of this plant medicine into her body, into her life.

Buhner next describes how he carefully introduced her to one drop of skunk cabbage tincture and slowly allowed it to affect her and move toward healing:

The power began to flow up into her lungs and out into the world. The old stagnant thing in her lungs began to flow with it, up and out of her body. The plant a channel, as I had been a channel. And interwoven with that moving stream was the living teaching, the medicine understanding of this plant, this ally, this living being that people call skunk cabbage.

If only all physicians could utilize this process with all of the patients who are struggling to free themselves of deep-seated suffering and approach healing at this depth.

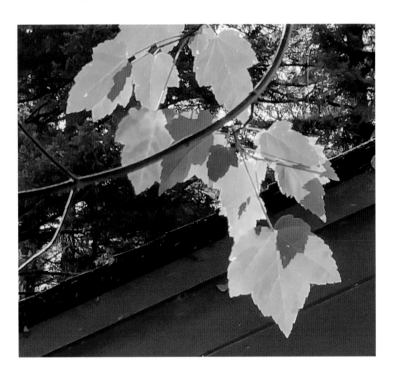

CHAPTER 16:

Medicine Men and Shamanic Healing: A Return to Our Connection to the Natural World

That Voodoo That You Do...So Well

I was fortunate to have had the opportunity to be exposed to Native American healing practices early in my medical training. As an intern at San Francisco General Hospital in 1971, one of my patients was a young Native American man who, in a bar fight, was knocked unconscious by a blow to the head from a cue stick. For four months he remained in a coma, unresponsive to all stimuli. The Native American community urged the hospital to allow a medicine man to perform a healing ceremony, and to our surprise, the hospital granted this request.

With outsiders banned from the room (except for nurses performing occasional vital sign checks), this young man was chanted and danced over, with drums and rattles accompanying the ceremony, for three days. Literally upon the completion of this ceremony, he suddenly woke up and wondered aloud, "Where the f—k am I?" This signaled his total recovery, and he left the hospital a few days later, following a battery of neurological tests showing that he had in fact fully recovered.

After I completed my internship, I began work with the Indian Health Service in Wagner, South Dakota. The small hospital there served a large area of the Sioux Nation in the southeastern corner of the state. To reinforce that my previous experience in San Francisco was not a fluke, a few months after I arrived in Wagner, a young Native American man was brought to us after suffering head trauma from a motor vehicle accident. Initially, he was sent to Yankton, our referral center, where the neurologists did all they could, but he remained in a coma and was sent back to our little hospital to recover closer to home. We cared for him for several months, but, like the first young man, he remained in a coma, unresponsive. The Sioux elders asked that a medicine man be allowed to perform a healing ceremony, and we readily agreed, as we had little else to offer.

Once again, after three days of chanting and dancing to the beat of drums and rattles, the young man woke up at the conclusion of the ceremony and uttered the very same words: "Where the f—k am I?" He, too, was able to leave the hospital the next day, fully recovered.

Coincidence? Perhaps, but unlikely. Having witnessed these events, I realized that conventional medicine might not have all of the answers, and that we should be open to other healing traditions and what they may offer us in the way of understanding and expanding the recovery process.

Intrigued by these experiences, I seized the opportunity to study herbal components of Native American healing with a local medicine man, John Fire Lame Deer, who co-authored the book *Seeker of Visions*, which was published in 1972, the year I arrived in South Dakota. John shared a number of his experiences with me, but my favorite humorous memory is the day he came into the clinic with a cough. When I naively asked him why he wasn't using some of the local plants to heal himself, he looked at me as if I was an idiot and said, "Why would I do that when you can give me penicillin?" It helps to put things into perspective.

I have pursued the study of healing from as many angles as possible, and following these early positive experiences, I read with great interest the anthropologist Michael Harner's book *The Way of the Shaman* when it came out in 1980. Harner studied a wide array of shamanic healing practices and realized that they shared a common thread. These practices usually involved the use of drums or other sounds, which enhanced the state of consciousness that allowed spiritual experiences to occur. In some cultures, chanting or mantras were used to the same effect. Once both the patient and the healer achieved a state of relaxation, allowing a deeper connection between them, the shamanic practitioner would sense clues from the patient as to the direction that healing needed to take place and would follow it wherever it might lead. Harner began to offer experiential workshops soon thereafter, and a physician friend and I went to one held in Chicago.

After explaining the basics of shamanic healing, Harner gave the attendees the opportunity to partake in several of these ceremonies. The one that stood out most to me is called the "spirit canoe." Picture thirty people in a fairly small area directed to seat ourselves on the floor in two rows (forming the outer rims of the "canoe") with Harner at the rear beating a drum. We were instructed to lock our arms around the person in front of us and lean back against the person behind us. I realized immediately that this position was really uncomfortable for my back, which began to ache, and I remember hoping that we would soon be shifting consciousness because I wasn't sure how long I could hold that position. Using guided imagery, which consisted of picturing ourselves to be traveling through spiritual water in a canoe, we were encouraged to simply notice what we "saw" as Harner took us along our journey, which lasted over an hour. I was relieved that, somehow, I forgot about my discomfort. At no time were we given instructions to visualize a particular animal or event.

After the completion of this ceremony, Harner instructed us to go off by ourselves and write down what we "saw" along the journey. I recall that I had the perception of seeing deer, elephants, and tigers. I had no idea what this meant, but when we regrouped to discuss our experiences, I was astonished to learn that all of the observers on my side of the "canoe" had seen the exact same set of animals! The participants on the other side had seen a different set, but all agreed that they had seen the same animals. The cohesion of that experience for all of us was remarkable to me.

After the workshop, my friend and I continued to study and prepare. The next stage of our training was to find our "spirit song." To do that, we decided (living in northern Minnesota) to go to the Boundary Waters and seek our songs in a pristine wilderness area. We took our canoes (real ones), portaged our way across many lakes, and made camp on a pretty little island in the middle of one. We created a small structure to serve as a kind of sauna to purify ourselves for this ceremony by heating up rocks and placing them in a pit in the earth that served as a floor for the tent, then pouring water over the rocks until we were sweating profusely. We meditated, cleared our minds, and then, to "receive" our special songs, called the spirits by playing our drums and using our rattles in the way we had been taught.

What happened next was overwhelming, frightening, and unexpected. The spirits came. Lots of them. Although their presence felt benign, it felt like we were being crushed by their weight. What were we thinking? With no expert guidance (our first mistake), we summoned who knew how many thousands of spirits that were hanging out in the Boundary Waters. Overwhelmed by what we had done, we crawled into our sleeping bags inside our tent and basically hid, cowering, until we felt that we were alone again. Fools rush in where angels fear to tread.

The takeaway from this was very clear: We were messing with energies we had no business tackling without experienced guides, and perhaps this was not our true path. We put aside our drums and rattles and pursued other studies. The experience was extremely powerful, however. If I'd had any doubts about the existence of "spirits" in the natural world, they were gone. And now I knew why the shamanic tradition entails a great deal of preparation and training under the guidance of someone who knows how to handle those energies.

PRAYER AND SPIRITUAL HEALING

Whether or not you accept the concept of evil spirits (or good spirits), what we are discussing, in essence, is the negative effects of certain energies and how to detect and ultimately remove them from another being.

Virtually every religion and native culture has some way of providing both a diagnostic and a treatment component, and all of these approaches share remarkable similarities. The Christian tradition includes many examples of faith healing with ceremonies that include prayer and the laying-on of hands for individuals and groups. I have had quite a few patients who were not improving with conventional treatment come back from such spiritual experiences healed, or nearly so, in very short periods of time.

The ability to feel energies is not limited to shamanic or religious practices. Since the perception of energy is a critical component of these practices, let's look at a few examples from other areas. Acupuncturists are trained to place their fingers over a patient's wrist to take their pulse and can enumerate over thirty different perceptions that enable them to feel energy blockages at different levels. They then use needles to direct the flow of those energies in ways that allow healing to take place.

Similarly (though not based in religion or native culture), osteopathic physicians are taught to feel a wide array of perceptions by placing their hands on a patient's body or head and correlate those perceptions with energetic blockages that they can shift and move with their hands.

Native healers are taught to perceive these energetic blockages in a variety of ways and to influence those same blockages with sound (chanting/drumming) and prayers. For instance, Tibetan sound therapies use specific chanted syllables to move energy through blocked areas of the body. Another example of sound therapy is given by Peter Levine, PhD, in the book *Clinical Applications of the Polyvagal Theory,* where he describes the process of chanting or singing "Vooooo" to reboot the vagus nerve when it is not functioning properly.

Seen from this perspective, prayer is an important component of healing, and it is underutilized in conventional medicine. Taken out of a religious context, at its essence prayer constitutes a positive visualization for some kind of positive outcome: healing, love, guidance, closure, or resolution of grief or anger, for example. I am also convinced that when prayers, or visualizations, are manifested by a group, the effectiveness of those prayers is magnified exponentially.

Central to this discussion is the idea that if the spirit is damaged, injured, or dysfunctional, it must be healed. Every culture has, in its own way, understood this and found ways of addressing it.

When I work with patients, I try to learn what spirituality means for them. Does it take the form of a religious practice or a desire to appreciate the natural world? What gives their lives meaning and purpose? Their answers influence the kinds of language that I use to communicate with them and the imagery I bring to mind to promote healing. For example, when working with someone who identifies as Christian or Jewish, I would talk to them in terms of God and prayer and being of service. For someone who is Buddhist, I would talk in terms of meditation and right action and speech. For a farmer, this might take the form of a discussion of the natural world or weather cycles. Each person should be approached from the deepest understanding we can gain of their belief system. With that in mind, we can use imagery and language that helps them relate to what they want to achieve in the form of healing.

While this chapter began with an attempt to move out of our comfort zone by discussing shamanic or native healing practices, I hope you can see that no matter what your beliefs, respecting and working with those beliefs is the most effective way to approach healing. We have much to learn about all of the different manifestations of energy, but using the ones that resonate with each individual patient will make our efforts more effective.

THE TEACHINGS OF PAUL GOODBERG

Last year, I was fortunate to be given the book *What Wants to Be Known* by Paul Goodberg. In it, Paul relates his experiences of learning healing techniques from three different sources.

First, he was trained in his grandmother's lineage of Central European healing. What makes his experience unusual is that no words were exchanged. All of the learning was done by careful observation, mimicking what the healer was doing, and receiving instruction via direct transmission, which means simply that the healer imparted what they were doing directly into Paul's consciousness.

Many people would come to Paul's grandmother's home, and she would help them to heal by utilizing several "gifts" that she would energetically impart. These gifts were handed down from generation to generation, primarily by the women in Paul's family. Having grown up in the presence of this healing, Paul acquired those gifts and was able to utilize them in the service of healing.

Later in life, he was drawn to Peru, where he was initiated into the Native healing culture over many years. Later still, he received healing gifts from the Mayan tradition.

Despite the disparate nature of these cultures, all teaching was done by direct transmission and in the form of gifts. Paul has spent time with many cultures in an effort to acquire as many gifts as possible so that he would be able to help as many people as possible. While much of his training was shamanic in origin, he does not think of himself as a shaman, but rather as someone who provides gifts for those who need them.

Intrigued by this book (which I encourage you to read for its fascinating account), I contacted Paul to see if he felt he could help me to become a better healer. It took time for both of us to decide that we were on the same page, but I have been studying with him twice a month for over a year now. I would like to share some of what I have learned and experienced, as I believe it is fundamental to the concept of what Native healing is about. Central to this type of healing is a deep communication with, and connection with, the natural world.

Following Paul's instructions, I am lying on my back on the ground in a small clearing near my home in the redwoods. As I look skyward, to my left are a small magnolia tree and a small olive tree. Surrounding me are towering redwoods. I am simply in contact with the Earth and await what wants to be known. To the best of my ability, I am not thinking about anything or doing anything— just experiencing the ground, the air, and the sounds of the forest. Almost every time I do this exercise, a raven comes around and caws at me or makes its typical clicking sounds. I do not know if it is acknowledging my presence or just being a raven and wishing I would not invade its territory.

I have been engaging in this practice several times a week for over a year. At first, I did not feel much, but over time I came to notice a warm, filling sensation in my hands, in a somewhat cyclical fashion, about every thirty or forty seconds. My hands fill with energy, and then the energy recedes into the ground. Paul tells me that I am finally feeling the "aliveness" of the Earth, and that sometime later I will feel an actual pulsation, which has healing properties and will help communicate with me. I will be patient.

Lying on my back looking up at the sky in my backyard at my redwood forest.

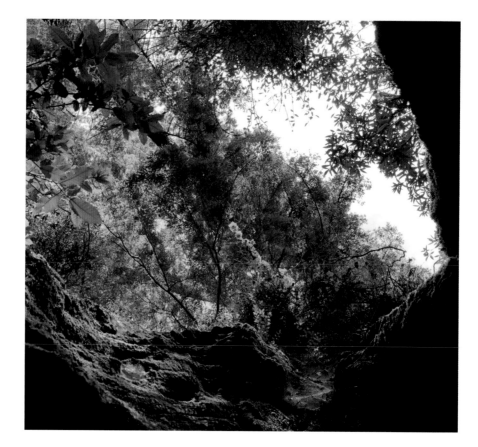

Recently, at the end of one of these sessions, I felt the presence of something ethereal, a being of some kind (the energy was benign and pleasant and felt a little like that of my wife, Cheryl) who knelt over me, placed some powdered herbs near my nostrils, and told me to breathe it in. When I took some deep breaths, I noticed a much stronger smell of the damp earth on which I was lying. Paul describes this as being visited by a "spirit" of some kind and says that I was given a gift "to further sensitize you at the level of smell." He noted that all such gifts are metaphoric and are intended to enhance communion with the natural world.

Several days later, I lay on the ground under a stump of a hollowed-out old-growth redwood tree on my property. Here, I felt my hands sinking into the earth more deeply and was surprised to notice that I felt strong breezes on my body, even though I was lying below ground level. At the end of this experience, I "heard" a disembodied "voice" (in my head) telling me, "Take care of my babies." Looking up, I noticed two second-growth redwoods not far away, but this stump was not part of a typical fairy circle (a name given to the many trees that grow around the base of a virgin redwood stump).

Paul tells me that, again, all gifts are metaphoric and that this communication did not mean that I take care of the visible trees, but to involve the entire forest. He feels that this was just the beginning of a connection to these woods, and over time, perhaps years, I will get a clearer message of exactly what "take care of my babies" means: what gifts I can give to the forest in return for the gifts that will be given to me.

As a result of these experiences, I am noticing several things. First, when walking on the headlands of my northern California coast, I am more and more aware of the vastness of the interaction between sky, sea, land, and sun. I am increasingly aware of how small I feel in that huge palette, but simultaneously I am part of it, one with it.

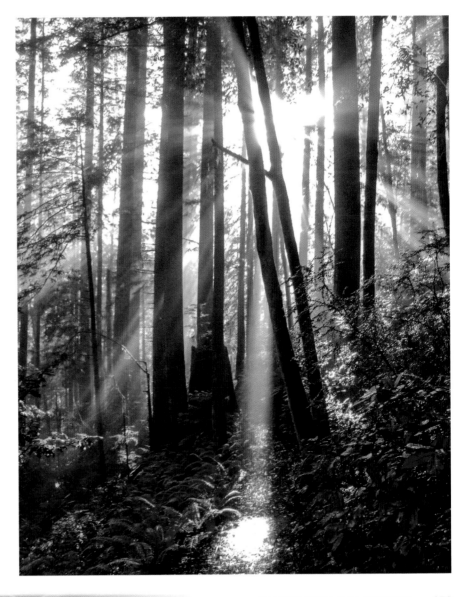

Stephen Buhner describes this so poetically on page 15 of *Plant Intelligence and the Imaginal Realm:*

> Time itself had changed, as if it were suspended—like the dust motes in the air.... I felt part of a living, breathing, aware, intelligent universe, and what is more...I felt wanted by that universe, as if I had come into the arms of my deepest and truest family. I felt at home in a way I never had before.

Perhaps the most profound example of Paul utilizing his healing gifts was a recent experience with my own health. In late January 2021, I began to have severe diarrhea and weight loss. I lost 37 pounds over the ensuing months and became weaker and weaker to the point that I could hardly walk or function. I sought medical care from many sources, but despite the caring and compassionate approach, it took months before I finally got the testing that showed I had a rare form of colitis, which included both major types, Crohn's disease and ulcerative colitis. I finally got into the hands of an excellent gastroenterologist who assured me that he had seen and successfully treated this type of colitis, but it would require some high-powered medications. I started intravenous infusions of Remicade and oral methotrexate, and within six weeks I was well on my way to recovery.

Given this context, in the early stages of my illness, I was surprised to find myself incredibly anxious and unable to do much of anything about this anxiety.

I was unable to think about anything but despair and doom. Although I have acquired many coping skills, including the ability to meditate, relax to a profound level, and let go of emotions that are affecting me, nothing I knew or did would help.

For over a month, I could not shake these intense feelings that had taken over me; I lived with doom and despair and fought it to no avail.

I finally called Paul and explained what was happening to me. After several sessions with his seeking and then finding the energetic block in my body, I experienced immediate and profound relief. That oppressive energy was instantaneously gone—just gone. Although at that time I was still undiagnosed, very ill, and losing weight, I was no longer in a panic about it. I was at peace with myself and with whatever would happen next. Although it took several more months to finally get the medical help I needed, the relief from this emotional state was a fabulous gift, and it allowed me to proceed with my medical care in a state of equanimity.

Whether connected to these experiences or not (I suspect it is), I have recently found myself "in the zone" for long periods of time. I suspect you will intuitively know what that phrase means, but let me expand on it to be clearer. A few examples:

Many years ago, while vacationing and working on Isla Mujeres, an island off the coast of Cancun, we met some friends whose daughter had just adopted a little puppy. She implored us, being an unusually adept saleswoman, to bring the puppy back to Missouri with us. I am not prone to doing things like this (but my wife is), so Cheryl was surprised when I asked her: "What about that puppy?"

Next came a series of amazingly copacetic events in which we literally were led to meet dozens of people who were to help us with this adoption process in a marvelous flow of connections. These next few days *felt* different from our normal waking days. Everything seemed to flow naturally, with no effort. As all of the pieces fell into place, every segue seemed magical. And so Kai (shown in the photo on the last page, with me, when we met him) came to live with us and become a mainstay of our lives. That, to me, is the epitome of being in the zone.

Another example of this energetic magic occurred during the last phases of writing my previous book, *Toxic*. I had completed most of the book, with only one or two chapters left to write, but I had not yet found a publisher and was uncertain how to proceed. Out of the blue, an individual sought me out, hoping I had a book he could publish. His vision for the book and mine were identical. We shared the same passion that this book had the capacity to help thousands of suffering patients, and together, we worked to create it. That publisher, Erich Krauss at Victory Belt, and the wonderful editor he provided to me, Pam Mourouzis, entered the scene exactly when I needed them, and the energy we all gave to that project was palpable. We were again in the zone.

What I am trying to describe here is that since I began studying with Paul Goodberg, I am, as I write these words, back in the zone. The unifying, connecting "rightness" of what I am doing feels different from my normal working activities. Ideas are flowing, connecting, joining. Driving my car, taking a walk, the steady stream of images and words is inspiring: I keep a pad and pen with me to write them down as they come, fast and furious, and at times I can barely keep up. But it is exhilarating and joyous and bursting with life.

I can't wait to experience the gifts I will receive next and see how I can use those in the service of healing.

Central to this type of healing is a deep connection with, and communication with, the natural world. As detailed in Stephen Buhner's description of how we can communicate with and learn from plants (see Chapter 15), we must remember that we, too, are a part of this planet that allows us to inhabit it, and it is critical to make every effort to honor that connection and re-establish that lifeline.

CHAPTER 17:

How to Find, Nurture, and Improve Your Intuitive Abilities

If you were secretly hoping that I would reveal to you, in this last chapter, some profound mystical truth, an incantation or mantra, perhaps, or a bit of arcane knowledge to magically bring you to enlightenment, I am sorry to disappoint you. My message here is a lot simpler but, for those who will be open to it, I hope just as meaningful.

Throughout this book, we have explored the importance of incorporating our perceptions of energy into medical diagnosis, and the ramifications of these perceptions. As I am sure is clear by now, I believe that every human being is born with the ability to perceive energy in many forms, but we all differ in our innate abilities to access these energies, with some types predominating and others in the background or hardly noticeable.

These perceptions are not limited to the practice of medicine, of course—that is simply the field that is most familiar to me. Attorneys, for example, also utilize some of these perceptions. (This is taken to a higher scientific form in the television show Bull, in which a psychologist utilizes an array of energy measurements to decide which potential jurors would be most likely to support the legal case at hand.) Scientists and inventors claim all kinds of insights as the source of inspiration for new ideas. So I don't think it is much of a stretch to suggest that if you were to spend some time enhancing these abilities, the effort would serve you well, no matter your occupation. Simply being able to "read" people better would improve all human communication.

In this final chapter of the book, I would like to briefly review how to do just that.

TRUST IS WHERE IT STARTS

You are constantly bombarded by energetic information. You don't really need to go looking for it. You are surrounded by it. In fact, your nervous system has been filtering all of these stimuli for you to bring to your attention what you have trained it to do. If you were unable to filter, or block, a great deal of these stimuli, you would risk being confused and distracted to the point that you would be unable to function. Schizophrenia is the embodiment of this problem. A person with schizophrenia is unable to shut down this barrage of stimuli and is overwhelmed to the point that they are, at times, unable to function. So it is clear that we need to have a filtering system in place to deal with the world we live in.

From infancy, you have been teaching yourself, at times with the help of others, which stimuli to pay attention to. We all have preferences. Some are positive and others are negative.

On the positive side, perhaps your family was musically oriented and you have been listening to music since childhood. Perhaps you learned to play an instrument or sing and have accordingly focused your perception on sounds that resonate with you. Those with special abilities in this realm are told they have "a good ear."

Perhaps your family loved books or films, and you are innately drawn to those areas. Perhaps they enjoyed some other form of art—drawing, painting, or ceramics—and your eyes are drawn in those directions.

Perhaps your family loved nature and spent many hours hiking, camping, bicycling, fishing, or hunting, and you are drawn to stimuli that evoke those memories.

Perhaps food was important in your family, and the aromas of cooking are what get your attention.

From these stimuli, you learned what to pay attention to in order to augment your feeling of enjoyment.

On the negative side, perhaps your family was prone to shouting or other loud noises. Perhaps they treated each other with silence. If alcohol was involved, you may have learned to recognize how to behave in such a way to minimize violence by "walking on eggshells." From these stimuli, you learned how to shut out or shut down your nervous system to take in as little of this negative energy as possible.

With each passing year, you modified your nervous system to maximize the stimuli that fed you and minimize the ones that you found unpleasant. What you probably did not realize is that by doing so, you were training your nervous system to make you comfortable by making certain things your areas of focus and, accordingly, ignoring other stimuli that may have been useful to acknowledge.

As children, it is essential that we do this filtering in order to survive. As we enter adulthood, we are largely unaware that we are no longer in survival mode, and we can deal with the stressors of life with a great deal more information and tools that we have acquired. The result is that we are capable of handling far more stimuli than we could as children, but we are often limited by our previous experiences. Unless we make a conscious effort to expand our coping abilities, we may be left with nothing but the coping mechanisms we resorted to as children in order to get by.

That's where trust comes in. First and foremost, we must learn to trust ourselves—to trust in our abilities to perceive correctly, sort through complicated information, and make good decisions to do what is in our own best interests. We will make mistakes. If we are open to learning from them and do not focus on blaming ourselves for those mistakes, by trial and error trust will grow.

The single most important quality in developing intuition and instinct is the growth of that trust. Your body is continuously picking up information, and as you begin to trust what your senses are telling you, your trust will grow. To some extent, this runs counter to our cultural predisposition to put the emphasis on what our brains can figure out. Our minds, exposed to rafts of conflicting information, are easily confused or misled. Our bodies are not.

Learning to trust our senses as a more accurate guide to this information is key. If your nose picks up a foul smell, it is a foul smell. Your mind can try to tell you that it has examined the area and found no source for this smell, but the fact that you are being exposed to a foul smell remains unchanged. Your mind is telling you, "There is no reason to move," while your nose is telling you, "Get out of here!"

The more attention you pay to what you are feeling, the more accurate your perceptions will be. Over time, you will begin to find that you can count on these perceptions to guide you through the difficult choices you face. You will begin to notice that when you relied on your mind for answers, sometimes those answers were good and sometimes they were misleading. When you relied on your feelings for answers, you were much better informed.

As you begin to trust those feelings, you will also discover that you are getting much more information—reliable information—which will be of use to you in perceiving the world. A simple example is the adage, "Judge people by their actions, not their words." Charismatic individuals can use words to convince you to believe things that run counter to their actions. This is in the best interest of the charismatic who is influencing you with words, but not necessarily yours. This is one of the central tenets of advertising—convincing us with words or pictures that we need something we don't.

Counter to this are the quiet individuals who do not say much and do not promote themselves, but are always doing good things: helping elderly neighbors, participating in charity drives, contributing to the community. Their deeds speak for themselves.

This is especially true for trust as it applies to intuition and instinct.

The more you trust yourself, the more you will find yourself allowing information into your nervous system in various ways: you may see pictures, hear phrases or words, or feel sensations that seem to come from "out of the blue." You will discover that this information is of great value almost all the time and needs to be honored. As you come to appreciate what you are picking up, you will increasingly trust this information, and you will be on your way to an enhanced relationship with the world as you know it. It will open up for you, expanding into greater possibilities of communication, interaction, and appreciation.

It starts with trust.

IMPROVING INTUITION

There are dozens of books out there that will walk you, step-by-step, through the process of enhancing your intuitive gifts. That is not what this book is about. It is not about technique, or method, or following steps. While those approaches are fine, I have concerns that following these techniques makes you prone to relying on technique rather than your own perceptions.

The process I am arguing for is both simple and very complicated. To enhance your gifts requires being completely present in the moment so that you optimize the possibility of connecting energetically with people, animals, plants, and the natural world. On the surface, it sounds simple: just be present. However, it turns out that it can be very difficult to get out of our heads, our thoughts, and our preconceived ideas and to get fully into our bodies to be present. Doing so requires dedication and patience without expectation, and this is not an easy place to enter.

To emphasize the importance of fully embracing our sensory experiences, let me recount a recent dream. In the dream, I am participating in a workshop for osteopathic physicians who are studying cranial work, and some of the advanced students tell me that what I am feeling is the idea of the perceptions we are studying, not the perceptions themselves. I am saddened by the realization that these advanced students are aware that I am not fully experiencing the energetic perceptions we are trying to master, but at the same time am aware that they are correct. I wake up with the understanding that I need to stay with the perceptions I am taking in from the patient I am treating until I feel them more completely, more intensely, so that I can then transmit healing to the patient at a more profound level.

To reiterate, the more open you are to fully experiencing and becoming a part of the sensory world in which you live, the more it becomes a part of you and begins to share with you.

Intrinsically, attempting this sort of openness can be frightening. In a world that can be filled with stress, and even danger or evil, I suggest you find a safe place in which to allow yourself to open up. There are some disturbing energies out there—but there are incredible connections as well, and to maximize your ability to be alive, I hope you will take the risk.

In many books, authors refer to this process as becoming a "spiritual warrior." It took me many years to understand the word *warrior* in this context because I could not associate the concept of fighting with opening. I am now beginning to realize that *warrior* simply refers to having the courage to allow this opening to occur and to trust that it will bring about spiritual and emotional benefits. So, in this sense, I hope you will become a warrior and manifest the courage to take this journey.

As I discussed in the Preface to this book, doing so is especially important now, as we face the devastating effects of the COVID-19 pandemic. Our efforts to protect ourselves and our families and friends from exposure to COVID—maintaining prolonged separation from others, keeping our distance or isolating ourselves completely, and wearing masks at all times—have had a profound effect on our consciousness. We are literally experiencing global PTSD. It is imperative that, as the pandemic subsides, we begin to let go of this fear, this separation, this distancing, and reconnect at the deepest level possible with our loved ones and the natural world, which are our sources of connection.

To heal from this awful experience requires an awareness of the fact that we all are in need of healing. We cannot simply go back to what we think we remember about what life was like before the pandemic hit; we have to consciously work on letting go of this fear we have carried and embrace life again wholeheartedly. Otherwise, we are looking at decades of protracted isolation, and we are setting ourselves up for harm from those who would take advantage of our fears.

Over the course of my life, I have attempted to acquire what spiritual wisdom I could derive from studying many traditions. In my own way of distilling this information, I have come to believe that a spiritual life, well lived, consists of three major ingredients:

- BE GRATEFUL.

- BE PRESENT.

- BE OF SERVICE.

COVID-19 and the constant media attention it has engendered have attempted to take over our consciousness. If we can be aware, as often as possible, of the gifts and blessings we already have, we can let go of that fear and remember the beauty and goodness that still predominate in this world. In order to do so, we need to be present to it, mindful of it, as often as we can. Remembering to breathe deeply and fully gives us the opportunity to become more aware of not only what is going on around us, but what is occurring in our own bodies right now.

We can let go of these oppressive tensions and focus on what is meaningful to us in the here and now. And by trying our best to be aware of the suffering of those around us and be of service to them, we can get out of our own negative thoughts and increasingly understand that we are not alone. Many, many other beings are experiencing difficulties as well. Reaching out to them takes us away from our internal dialogues, and we become more connected to the whole world and can feel, again, our part in it.

Remembering our birthright of being a part of the natural world is our way out of this situation, and it's the key to understanding how we can heal. Trusting our perceptions and tuning in to our gifts are central to moving forward, and I hope that these words will encourage you to undertake this journey.

EPILOGUE

THE EMBODIMENT OF NEILNESS

I am walking down a country road not far from my home. It is a walk I take often while trying to experience the beautiful world around me—sunshine, blue sky with a few scattered clouds, redwood trees, some scattered houses. I like to feel this world with my whole body rather than take it in through my eyes and analyze it (my usual way of perceiving it). Trying to feel the sky, the clouds, the earth, the trees, the whole of it, in my body. Opening up my senses to it: The silence, at times, is deafening. The smells of wet earth, fresh rain, and a hint of mushroom, and feeling the sun upon my face is easier than taking in the totality of this experience. The breath of wind has a cool nip.

In a sense, I am attempting to emulate how my dogs take this same walk. Although I have no idea how dogs really feel, my pets seem to embark on this walk with fresh eyes and noses sniffing the air, excited about this adventure as if we had not done this walk hundreds of times before. They appear to be far better at coming to this experience with what I am looking for: beginner's senses.

My mind keeps wandering, and I make the effort to stay in my body to attempt to feel this whole experience, whatever comes, with every step. I am not very good at it, but I keep trying.

Almost everything I read these days seems to urge me to get out of my head and into my body. That is how I can really experience this lovely world that I live in; and the natural world will help to keep me healthy, connected, and inspired. With a little luck, I can bring that sense of embodiment to my work with patients, my teaching, and my beloved family.

This is a part of the message I have hoped to impart in this book. To embrace our birthright of energetic connectedness, love, generosity, and kindness, we need to embrace our neglected relationship with the natural world. To do so is to be truly alive and to be aware of the aliveness of the earth, sky, sun, moon, ocean, trees, and all life forms on our planet. I know that this connection is dissolving, and I worry we do not understand that this connection is our lifeblood. Without it, where and what will we be?

I hope that my children and grandchildren will seek and embrace this connection, and that you will, too. The future of our planet depends on it. If this book has, in any way, reminded you of these truths, then it has been worth the effort for me to write it.

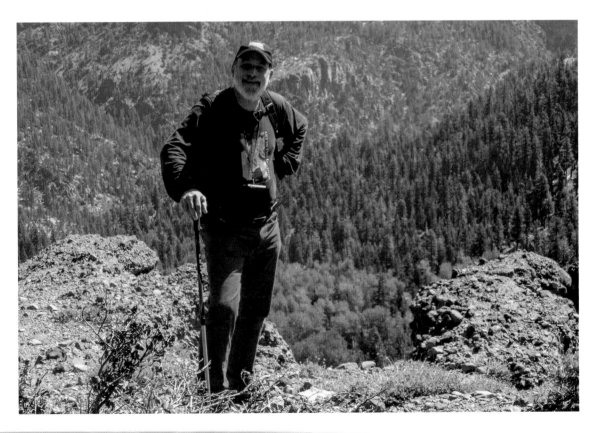

ACKNOWLEDGMENTS

I suspect that every book written is, to some extent, a labor of love, and this one is no exception. It takes a team of dedicated people with different talents to bring this to fruition.

First, I want to thank Pam Mourouzis, my amazing editor, for taking my manuscript and bringing it into existence. It is a wonderful experience to be in such close sync with a woman with such vision. I also want to thank the entire team at Victory Belt, and especially my publishers, Erich Krauss and Lance Freimuth, for their continuing support.

I have been blessed, throughout my life, to meet incredible teachers in every field, so I thank T. T. Liang, Stuart Olson, Abraham Liu, and Gary Stier, my tai chi teachers; Ginny Morgan and the staff of Spirit Rock for their instruction in meditation; and James Jealous, DO (who unfortunately left us this year), Edna Lay, DO, and Louis Hasbrouck, DO, for their sharing of their knowledge of osteopathic medicine and healing.

For my dear, departed friend Stanley Weisenberg, who shared our adventures in Yosemite, and for Rod and Jo, who owned the Sea Rock Inn in Mendocino and taught me the art of dowsing in the early 1970s, so many thanks. Gratitude also goes to Doug Hiza, MD, who joined me in pursuit of shamanism in the 1980s.

Special thanks go to Paul Goodberg, who has taught me and healed me, and to Stephen Buhner, the brilliant herbalist who has shared so much of his knowledge of plants and healing.

Of course, I am truly grateful to all of the wonderful healers who have contributed to this book: Judy Tsafrir, MD, Gene Nathan, MD, Carolyn McMakin, DC, Dave Ou, MD, Jeffrey Greenfield, DO, Joel Friedman, MD, Sonia Rapaport, MD, and Emily Rowe, MD, for bringing their experiences and knowledge into the context of our book.

It may be a cliché (although, like most clichés, there is a great deal of truth in it), but this book would not have been possible without the incredible support and love given to me by my wife, Cheryl; my two adorable puppies, Sasha and Eddie; my children, Aviva, Jules, and David; and my grandchildren, Avi, Angeli, and Wilder.

As always, I am eternally grateful to all of my thousands of patients and wonderful colleagues, who over the years have trusted me, supported me, and taught me with open hearts and minds. Thank you!

INDEX